Lust For Living

By John B. Lust

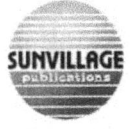

www.sunvillagepublications.com

Personality…and the Body
By J.H.Effenberg, Ph.D.

Copyright © 2010

No part of this publication may be reproduced, stored in a retrieval system or transmitted in any form or by any means, electronic, mechanical, photocopying, recording or otherwise, without prior written permission from the publisher.

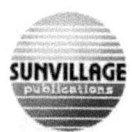

www.sunvillagepublications.com

Cover photography by Winthrop Brookhouse
Cover design by www.WebCopyAlchemy.com

For more powerful self-help techniques
and mind-tools visit us online at:
www.MindPowerSelfHelp.com

Dedicated to the memory of

DR. BENEDICT LUST

who made America aware of
NATURE'S healing power

TABLE OF CONTENTS

CHAPTER   PAGE

1. YOU ARE, BEING REBORN

 Y OU ARE being reborn!

If you believe that a power lies within the secrets of nature, that great knowledge can bring you new health and life, then this book is for you!

If you understand that man's opposition to nature, his ignorance of the laws of life, have deprived you of health and life, then too, this book is for you!

If you are willing to cast out the errors and misinformation of your earliest years and learn anew the ways of natural living, then life can begin again for you and "old age" can become a useless, meaningless phrase. For with new knowledge and determination, you can truly say, "I AM BEING REBORN!"

From this moment on, your life can take on a fuller meaning than it has ever held for you; with each page you read, you can expand the horizons of your existence beyond the reaches of your dreams—to a scope you never knew existed. Equipped with this new understanding of yourself and your world, you can go forth to build a healthiness and physical purity that can defy the years themselves. You can do this—if you desire it. The choice is yours!

These are not hastily written, ill-considered promises. I do not hold lightly the responsibility of these words, any more than I would expect you to. Human life is far too precious, too wondrous a thing for any man to deal with in promises and pretenses. The words you now read have been some twelve years in the contemplation and writing.

In 1940, at Yungborn Sanitorium, in Florida, I began the compilation of the notes and data that were to form the basis of this book. I worked for three years under the guidance of my life-long friend and uncle, Dr. Benedict Lust, as together we gathered material for what we believed would be the most complete and comprehensive book in the field of natural therapy. After three years of intensive work, I entered into the final rewriting of that book. And then tragedy struck! Yungborn Sanitorium was burned to the ground.

The Sanitorium was packed to capacity with the many souls who had come to us for rest and physical repair. The hours that followed the horrible realization that the Sanitorium was ablaze were filled with the hectic work of saving the patients who had bedded down for the night. Time and again, we raced back and forth from that inferno to carry our human cargoes to safety. Twice Dr. Lust's clothes and hair caught fire, and it was necessary to beat out the flames. What I did not realize then was that the injuries he had suffered in that blaze were soon to bring death to my uncle, Dr. Benedict Lust, who, at the age of seventy-three, was the most vital and hard working person I had ever known, or have known to this day.

In the end, the Sanitorium was burned to the ground, and there was more than one immediate casualty from that fire. In the confusion and horror of that night, I had forgotten the library, in the rear of the building, where, in a large oak desk, the original notes for this book were burned to a crisp.

In the years since that awful night, I have spent much of my working time recreating the pages that were lost to flame. Without the immediate guidance and friendly reassurance of Dr. Lust, it has been no simple task. And I can only say in honesty that this book would never have been possible were it not for those many years of close association with the most creative thinker in the history of natural therapy.

What I have brought to these pages is the wisdom of many years and many men, least among them myself. But what you find in this book is only that which you are willing to seek out. Your future life is what you are willing to create with your own brain and hands. The evil done to men is done by men. The good that can undo that evil must also be done by men. And it is important to remember that nothing is bought cheaply, neither happiness nor unhappiness.

Health! Years of painless, joyful existence that have been but a dream until this moment. If you will but pay the small price, a price of conviction, self-honesty and loyalty to your new life, all these can be yours:

Happiness! The wondrous feeling of being at peace with yourself, the earth and all mankind. The happiness that comes with understanding your place in life; your part in the scheme of earth, trees, rivers and man which we call our world!

Longevity! Decades and decades of a good life, a bold and glowing existence that can be yours, with the understanding and conviction to make it so.

To each his own desires! Color your hopes, your dreams, your aspirations with the ripe tones of reality, then multiply them by the number of dreams you have never dared to dream.

THIS IS THE PROMISE OF YOUR REBIRTH!

A tall order? Of course. Impossible? Only the way something you have never attempted seems impossible before the doing.

To want to be, that is not enough. To know how to be, that is too little. To *want,* to *know how,* to *determine to be,* that is the way of all successful men. Primary to all of these is self-honesty. You can cheat others, now and then. You can rarely cheat yourself. You can *never* cheat nature!

Many years ago, Dr. Albert Rutsen Allen, a man for whom I have always had deep admiration, taught me a fundamental rule of living. Dr. Allen was one of those successful men who could take a great truth and embody it in a simple physical action that, once seen, could never be driven from the mind. This day, I recall that he was holding a small wooden box in one hand and some pencils in the other. He pointed to the pencils.

"Count them," he said. I did, and found that there were four. He placed the pencils in the box, pretended to make some magic motions of his hand and then reopened the box. When he removed the pencils, there were now five!

"You tricked me," I said. "There were only four when you started." Dr. Allen laughed good-naturedly.

"Remember that," he said. "Don't forget it as long as you live. You can't get more out of life than you put in it. If you think you can do it, you're tricking yourself!"

I have never forgotten that. You must never forget it either!

You will gain from life only to the degree that you bring something to it. You will learn from this book only what you are willing to put into practice. If you reach a point in the reading in which some plan or exercise *is* outlined, and I suggest you try this out, then that is what I mean — now, today. Or, as the French entertainer, Chevalier, would say, "Not tomorrow, not ze next day, but r-r-i-i-ght *now!"*

When you reach a passage that says, "Recall from your own life," then stop reading long enough to do just that. What you yourself have experienced you will find hard to deny to yourself. Each time that you and I can reach a point of mutual experience, a true point of personal contact, we are coming closer to the kind of understanding that will make this book a part and working detail of your new life.

Beyond the personal dreams which each of us will bring to this new life, what do we mean by rebirth? Getting more out of life? Yes. That is only part of the story,. A release from many of the physical pains and mental anxieties that plague the average person? That, too, but again, this is merely a fraction of your new life. If you combine these two factors, a more productive life and a less painful and confused one, you find that between the two a third force is introduced. The absence of pain and anxiety increases your ability to create new values, while those new values which you create in turn increase your immunity to pain and anxiety. This is not a quantitative change but a qualitative one. "What we have produced from the combination of increased creativity and decreased depression is what we shall call *the force of life.*

Even with the *force of life* guaranteed us, we would still lack one important factor for genuine rebirth. Longevity! "What good is this new life if it is to be snatched from us? Must men be constantly cheated of the wonders of a long life? No!

Long life is possible! Longevity is desirable!

Men have denied themselves the full span of life through one terrible error. They have attempted to live without the natural source of life, nature! Men of science who would extend our life span, have made the same error in their work. They have tried to correct the error only to repeat it. They rejected nature. In the end, their work was rejected *by* nature! "The book of Nature is that which the physician must read; and to do so he must walk over the leaves." (Paracelsus).

Compare man's existence with that of other forms of life and you will see what we have done to ourselves in our constant tamperings with natural living. The natural life span of a dog is some twelve to fourteen years. A dog reaches full maturity within two years. Thus the natural life span of a dog is five to seven times the period required for maturity. Now if we multiply the period required for full human maturity (some twenty years), by the number seven, we arrive at the astounding figure of ONE HUNDRED AND FORTY YEARS!

Other animals, such as the turtle and certain birds, have been known to have *actual* lifespans of one hundred to three hundred years! In any number of living things, time and again we arrive at that same formula of longevity, SEVEN TIMES THE PERIOD OF MATURITY!

This is the promise of nature. This is what human longevity should be. We, being far above the order of other animals, have enough intelligence and understanding to make even that figure an underestimation of man's final fulfillment. We could do this, if we would learn one simple, all-powerful truth. *We are the creation of nature!*

Creations of nature, we must live in harmony with nature. Having realized that, and when you have accomplished it, you can know the full promise of life. You can apply the rule of seven and make present life-spans seem like childhood beside that of your new life.

Can it be done? It has been done! It is being done now!

On earth now, in various isolated and out-of-the-way areas of our globe, there are people who count their lives not in years, but in decades. People are living today who were alive at the time of Louis Napoleon, seventy-five years before the radio tube was invented. "Where are they?" you ask.

Let us rise to the high peaks of the Himalayas, or the broad, plain lands of China. From here, fabulous and documented tales return to us of natural life-spans averaging one hundred and ten, one hundred and twenty years! It is doubtless for this reason that authors like H. Rider Haggard and James Hilton chose just such remote areas for the scenes of their novels, "SHE" and "LOST HORIZONS," books dealing with a people who counted their lives in *centuries!*

These areas of long life are being closely investigated today. Scores of scientific teams from many lands are living among these people, documenting their histories, studying their lives.

It is particularly important to you that these men have centered their investigations around three major factors: diet, soil and living habits.

We want to know more about what these people eat, what they wear, how they live. Because we realize now that which Benedict Lust proclaimed more than half a century ago. "Tell me what a man eats and how he treats his body, and I will tell you how long that man will live!"

Diet, yes. Living habits, of course. Why the soil? `Why are these scientists investigating the earth upon which these people live? They are learning that soil is the mother of life. Earth feeds tree. Tree feeds fruit. Fruit feeds man. Here is the prime example of nature's cycle. It is this great cycle which offers us relief from pain; health through natural living. This kinship of earth, plant and man is the secret of life!

Why is it that we, who have advanced so far in one hundred years, must turn to the so-called backward peoples to understand the secrets of longevity? Why, with our theories of medicine, physics, chemistry, food processing, why do we die at the prime of life—while half-way around the earth, in primitive villages, men live twice our years? They look like us, possess the same organs and tissue as we do. Then, if all men are created alike at birth, what has happened to these people since birth that has made possible their wonderful century of life? One thing, primarily: these people have never lost their place in nature's cycle.

They rise with the sun. Do you? They live largely on vegetables and fruits from organic gardens (grown without the use of unnatural agents). Do you? Bread is made from dark whole grains. They eat sugar in its natural form, when they eat it at all, not the white refined stuff we use to sweeten our food. They bathe naturally, in open streams. They sleep without the aid of drugs and walk without the use of shoes. How many of these things do you do? How many could you do?

If you can say that you actually and regularly practice even two of the above, then you have a higher score than most men of modern society. Most people practice none! Many because they do not understand the meaning and importance of these seemingly unrelated matters. Others because they feel it would be too "uncomfortable," too "unconventional" in a modern society. You see how we have twisted our lives around. We have brought ourselves to the point where we consider that which is natural to be unnatural, and that which is removed from nature to be the true way of life. Is it any wonder that ours is the era of heart disease, cancer, constipation, goiter, chronic indigestion, allergies, ulcers and constant fatigue, colds and headaches? If we defy nature, can we expect nature to refuse that defiance? We may hope so, but nature will not. Our choice is clear.

You may live with nature, in health, in the joy of full life, in the long years of natural existence. Or you may make enemies of nature, opposing the will and the patterns of nature, living in pain and dying before your time!

Must you live as these people of the mountains and plains of the northern lands do in order to be *in.* harmony with nature?

Of course not. Because some people have misunderstood and believed that living in harmony with nature is some sort of "caveman" movement, they have foolishly rejected their re-birth.

It is possible to live with nature, observing the laws of the earth, and to remain citizens of our modern civilization at one and the same time. Wherever you live, whether in the streets of the city or the rural lanes of the country, you can maintain all the comfort and ease of your present existence and still live in harmony with the laws of nature.

Your re-birth demands that you reject only that which is harmful within your present existence. Modern living offers great conveniences. Nature offers life itself. There is a meeting place between these two. We can find that meeting place together. "Come forth into the light of things, let Nature be your teacher." (Wadsworth).

The past one hundred years have been years of great enlightenment. Unfortunately, that wisdom has been largely in the direction of improving the body comforts without a like understanding of the improvement of the body itself. Even while we have busied ourselves in learning the fundamental laws of chemistry, physics, electricity, we have been learning about man and his relationship to the earth he lives upon.

Doubtless our most important discovery in the past one hundred years is the knowledge that man is a part, a glorious part of nature. Nature's pattern, above all else, is motion. Constant motion. A never-ending cycle of change, Electricity, as we now understand it, is motion. The universe is motion. Man himself is motion. Understand this, for it is basic in understanding yourself and your new life.

Though you may hear the same name and return to the same house both evenings, you are, on Tuesday, a different person from the one you were on Monday. Twenty-four hours have wrought change; subtle change, true, but change none the less. You are a day apart from the one you were.

Think back, for one moment, to the people around you who are important to you and your life. These are the people you know best. Think now of the changes within their lives; not the dramatic overnight changes which writers of fiction like to dwell upon. I refer to the everyday motion and the direction of that motion which has brought them from where they were five years ago to this present point in time. It is fundamental to living. Without this day-to-day motion, your life would be static and re-birth would be impossible!

That is why it is so important for you to understand. Each day brings changes, both mental and physical. Your body is constantly changing. Are you aware of it? If not, then learn it now, for you are about to apply this knowledge and change your life—mind and body!

Look at your hand. Turn it in the air, examine it closely. Is it the same hand you had yesterday, a year ago, ten years ago? It *is* not! In twenty-four hours, since this time yesterday, a small area of your hand has been shed and new tissue has replaced it. Overnight a bit of you has been reborn. This is constant, never-ending. New tissue replaces old. You scrape your arm and it bleeds. Within a matter of days, that scraped skin has been naturally removed and new skin has replaced it.

Every organ, every bone, every single cell of life you call your body is in the endless process of change. A single red blood corpuscle has a life span of two months. This means that, in a period of 60 days, every blood cell you had at the beginning has done its work and ceased to exist, while new cells have been born to replace them all. This is the hope, the root of re-birth.

Your body is essentially a different body from that which you possessed ten years ago. New organs, blood and skin have all been reborn in a period of seven years. Grasp this fact. Understand it and understand how it applies to your own life. What can it mean to you? What can it mean to the dream of a long and creative life?

When a mold has been cast, it cannot be changed. It can be junked or it can be used, whether fit or unfit for the work it was intended. A ball of clay is another matter. We shape it once. If we are not satisfied with the results, we smooth out a little piece here, remove a bit there and replace it at another point where it will do the most good. Clay is malleable, capable of being shaped and reshaped. So are we! Brain, bone and mind can be reborn either through the creation of new tissue, or as in the brain, through retraining, rejecting the errors of the past and learning anew each moment of our lives. "Nature shows the true and perfect way, so learn how never from her paths to stray." (Adolf Just)

It is strange how so many of us accept the law of constant motion in all things that concern us except that most important matter of all, our health and life. The housewife who finds her home cluttered with the dirt and waste of living, does not hesitate to clean it out weekly and maintain a neat and balanced household from day to day. She even sets aside one or two occasions during the year, generally Spring and Fall, when she cleans her house from top to bottom and creates a fresh, new atmosphere within her home. She knows that the dirt and decay of her household *is* not a "normal" and unchangeable condition, and she refuses to let it become so. She recognizes the law of constant motion and applies it to creating a wholesome atmosphere in her home.

But that same woman frequently loses this understanding when she concerns herself with her health and life. If she is overweight, she may accept this, using such foolish phrases as, "it's natural for me," or "that's the way I'm built." If she suffers from headaches or chronic indigestion, she reminds herself that her mother or father suffered similarly and therefore it cannot be prevented. "That's how my family is," she will say. In her own life, her own health, she has rejected the law of constant motion. She has forgotten that her body, like her home, can be cleared of waste and decay. She has neglected to apply the same logic to her own health as that which she applied when her home became disheveled. She has forgotten that life and health, like all things which confront us, are of our own making. What men have done, men can undo. This is the past history of man and the promise of a bright future.

Man is the living symbol of progress. He changes. He adapts himself to natural changes around him. He learns and applies his learning to making a better life for himself. Silk is too expensive? We'll invent rayon. Rayon is perishable? Let us find out how to make nylon. Nylon feels cold? Somebody discover orlon, please. That is what we have done since the beginning of time. We have done this everywhere *except* for health and life itself!

How much time, money and study has been invested in the discovery of what makes for a healthy body, a sound mind, a happy life? Pennies, as against dollars in comparison. And even these pennies have been spent in the pursuit of an understanding of health that brings us once more into direct combat with nature. Medical research is spent in discovering the so-called wonder drugs, which day by day prove less wonderful and more harmful to mankind than most physicians are willing to admit. How much time and money are we willing to spend in understanding the natural sources of health—sun, light, air, food, soil? The answer lies in the present state of our national health.

The longer we refuse to devote ourselves to an understanding of what makes for health, the greater the problem will become. Here, too, is a cycle. The man who *is* ill is the man who broods upon his illness. This despair in turn induces illness. The result is that modern man has lost great measures of the vital sense of existence. Joy is a product that is fast disappearing from the open market. The will to live is being sapped through despair, yet, " 'Tis very certain the desire of life prolongs it." (Byron).

No one can help a man who refuses lo help himself. If your life is to be a long and happy one, you must *want* to live! You must love life! If you want to be brought from despair into a hopeful and vital state of existence, it can be done by proving to yourself that there is much to live for. There is a whole beautiful, lovable and loving world to go on living in. Can you do that? Can you prove that life is really worth the price we pay for it? Can you add up your joys and sorrows and come out with a good chart? Or are you running in the red, with more debits of sadness and gloomy views than you have credits of happy experience, hope and faith in the future?

This is not just idle chatter. This is the substance of all that we have ever learned about health and rational living. If you cannot say, with certainty, that you want: to live—that you love life—then you are not prepared to build the kind of body and mind that will extend your life and end pain and disease.

If you know within you that life is precious, life is good, then more abundant health and happiness are yours for the building. If this is not so, then you have a job to do on yourself before you read another page of this book. It is not a long or difficult task. It is pleasant, to say the least. You will be repaid, in two short hours, with a new lifetime of happiness. Is it worth it? I believe it is.

Here then is what I ask of you and what you must ask of yourself. When you have come to the end of this page, put the book down for a while. Put on your hat and coat (unless the weather permits you to enjoy the outdoor world without benefit of outer garments.) Now step out of the house and look around you. Choose a direction you don't so often take. As you walk, breathe deeply. Enjoy the air for the wonderful tonic it is: tonic for body as well as soul. Breath is life! Breathe fully to live fully!

Look around you as you walk. See the homes you have never really seen before, though you may have passed them a thousand times. See the people who live within those homes. Watch them relaxing, working in their gardens, tinkering with their autos or playing with their children. Watch the children, particularly. There is the future! In those children you see tomorrow. How does that future look to you—dim? No, it does not! Their laughter, the serious little faces they wear as they work out a boy or girl-sized problem, the joy in their songs, their shouts, their strong young bodies—you know that they are the promise of a bright tomorrow.

Man is only one of nature's great works. Man is the jewel of nature's workshop. All else is the setting for that gem. What a magnificent setting. You can feel it, touch it, breathe and taste it. Feel the breeze; the warm green zephyr of spring, the crisp brown breath of autumn, the cool white bracing wind of winter. Take a leaf into your hand and examine it. Science speaks of plants as the simplest life form; so simple, they say. Yet man has never duplicated even this "simple" creation of nature. For here, in the smallest leaf, is the whole great power of life.

Look at the trees around you. What do you see? You see within the beech or evergreen a life-span of over one thousand years! There are cedar trees which live 700 years; chestnut and oak with a life-span of 2,000 years; cypress and yew that have lived 3,000 years, fifty times the so-called normal life-span of man. Near Athens there stands the famous olive tree of Plato that is more than two thousand years old. Yes, a tree that was born before the coming of Christ still stands today!

As if the above were not amazing enough, there are recorded claims of dracaena, tropical trees, that have lived for eight thousand years! These simple trees! Perhaps man could do with a good share of this simplicity. For of all these, cedar, chestnut, oak, cypress, olive and dracaena, there is one common factor: all live *with* nature, not against it! Man, who thinks that he can change the patterns of life without harm to himself, spins out his life in sixty-odd years and shakes his head in wonderment. But there are some men, and their legions grow with each passing day, who have learned to live in harmony with nature. If you would live the long and full life that all men desire, then you must make yourself a part of those who live the balanced life, the natural life. "Life is amply long for him who orders it properly." (Seneca).

This is the beginning of your road back to life. It is a road of friendship, health and joy. Here is where you will find the promise of real happiness.

Stop being a stranger to the world! Know the world, as well as all creations of nature, and you will see life for what it truly is: beautiful, warm, alive with every breeze, each ray of sun, each drop of rain. This is worth living for! It is there for us all.

The will to live! That is the key to the first day of your new life!

II. THE FIRST THREE STEPS OF YOUR NEW LIFE

"Mother Nature is the Great Bookkeeper. The day you are born, the books are opened and the balance has begun. From that moment on, every step you take, each morsel of food, ray of sunshine, breath of air is recorded, in your favor or against it. You may fool yourself, but no one fools the Great Bookkeeper!"

—Dr. Benedict Lust.

Mrs. D. M. was a woman of fifty-five. She was some forty pounds overweight. Her diet consisted largely of fat meats and starchy vegetables. She liked to indulge her appetite in creamy chocolates and rich desserts. Her life was spent indoors, and even vacations found Mrs. M. beneath a parasol, behind a newspaper, covered by long, neck-tight dresses and billowy hats. She died following a siege of pain and disease. What killed Mrs. D. M.? Which sunless day? Which foul-aired room? Which pound of chocolates?

Your human body *is* a marvel of construction. It is strong, resilient, capable of withstanding amazing amounts of abuse— but not endless abuse. Disease, decay and early death are not the products of any single excess or failure. Rather, they are the end result of living contrary to the laws of life day after day. The disease of the forties or fifties results from the mistakes of the twenties and thirties.

How must you begin your new life? What laws of nature must you start to observe with the first day of your re-birth?

The first day of your new life must begin with an onslaught against the enemies of your body and brain. For your body and mind are as much a part of one another as are tree and leaves. They cannot be maintained in separate conditions of health.

Therefore, the first day of your new life must begin with two primary conditions for longevity; painless existence and happy living.

1. You must believe in and be determined to achieve this condition of permanent good health by defeating the negative attitudes that have long been a part of your former life.

2. Even as you cleanse your mind of the negative thinking that would have removed happiness, health and years of existence from your life, you must cleanse your body of the toxins that you have been storing through the years. These are the poisons of decay, malnutrition, foul air, indoor life, to mention a few.

The basic prescription for natural living is a simple one. It consists of three functions which, once begun, must continue throughout the course of your new life if you are to live as nature intended.

1. CLEANSE BODY AND MIND; To combat the decay that unnatural existence has already brought to your body and mind, you must begin by cleansing yourself of the poisons of that life. By employing all the natural means of eliminating these toxins, a fresh and revitalized approach to life can be yours.

2. REPAIR THE DAMAGE: The toxins of unnatural life have wrought damage upon your body through the years. However, cleansing your body is not enough, if the or-

gans have already been damaged through dangerous, unnatural excesses and the absence of contact with nature.
Then you must proceed to rebuild the ravaged organs and
tissues of your body with careful application of nature's
agents.

3. MAINTAIN YOUR NATURAL HEALTH: Once
cleansed of toxins and with the ravages of unnatural existence repaired, you now can proceed to live in harmony
with nature, thus insuring the maintenance of your health
and happiness.

In outline form, these three laws of life seem simple enough.
But before you can even attempt to enforce this new discipline
upon your body, you must be sure that you understand all that is
involved.

There are four major exits for the waste matter accumulated
by your body. Most people are not aware of this. Certainly all of
us are aware of the pain and discomfort of constipation. The
bowel movement is a fundamental means of elimination, and the
corruption of this natural action spells more than discomfort for
the sufferer. Urination is, of course, the second most important
eliminatory action. There are two other means of elimination
which are important to the cleansing of our bodies and which are
too often overlooked by most of us. They are the exits of skin
and lung—perspiration and breathing.

Oxygen is a "nutrient," that is, a food. Your blood feeds upon
oxygen. Each organ, each cell of your body is revitalized by the
blood stream. Blood that is improperly fed cannot repair the
damaged tissues of your body. If the air you breathe is clean,
fresh, life-sustaining, then the blood will be properly fed. Your
breathing must eliminate every last remaining bit of exhausted

gas from the lungs and blood, so the blood system will not be forced to feed upon poisoned air.

I cannot stress too strongly that you must breathe deeply, so that exhalable gases will not be delayed in the lungs, and so that your blood will be fully saturated with oxygen. Breathe deep down to your abdomen, not high in your chest. You should remember that oxygen is an important nutrient and a substance that, by a process of oxidation, helps the organism not only to produce heat but also to get rid of the harmful, poisonous waste products of your metabolism.

The skin is possibly the most abused organ of elimination. Your body is covered with thousands of small openings called pores. Cleansed properly and permitted free access to sun, light and air, pores assist us in discarding waste matter from the system through perspiration and evaporation,. Denied air, sun and water, the decay of that waste will remain within your body, in part and upon the surface of your skin as putrified matter.

We might do well, while we are cleansing things, to start with our own kitchens. I cannot think of a better first step on the road to your new life than the one that leads us to your kitchen where we can proceed to cleanse the cupboards of dead food. Yes, dead food. Food that is devoid of life or life-giving elements. White sugar, white flour and processed cheese are three major offenders.

Sugar, natural or raw sugar, that is, is a good food. Sucked directly from the cane, it is a delightful food and you are missing something if you have never tasted sugar cane. The raw sugar extracted from the cane is a brown, pebbly substance that contains many natural minerals of value to the body. White sugar, granulated, powdered or even the refined brown sugar, which is not to be confused with the raw product, has no value to the human body other than the calories with which it supplies us. Since all foods that are high in caloric content and low in other nutrients, minerals and vitamins, are almost useless to us, it would be best to eliminate processed sugar from the diet altogether.

If your diet demands sweetening, and most of us have an active sweet tooth, then try raw sugar. A product called Grans, which is natural sugar, can be obtained at most grocery stores, and all special diet food shops, and will not only be beneficial to. you, but you will soon come to enjoy its tangy flavor far beyond that of the oversweet taste of refined sugar. Honey and molasses are also fine substitutes for refined sugar.

White flour is an even greater offender. "Wheat has often been called the staff of life, with its abundant supply of so many of the life-giving elements: vitamins and minerals. But white flour is an imposter. The heart of the wheat has been removed. The flour is processed and reprocessed to give it that snowy appearance that seems to spell goodness, and actually means uselessness. Here is another high-calory food that will sap energy from the body during digestion and add little more than fat to the system.

Dump that cannister of white flour now! Drop it in the garbage pail where it belongs. Fill the cannister instead with good, whole grain flour, which can be obtained at most grocers and any good diet food shop. The whole grain flour will provide you with energy, vitamins, particularly the B-complex, so important to health, and many of the required minerals.

Processed cheese cannot be called useless. It has a use. It is a fine means of encouraging constipation, if that is considered a use. Beyond that, the processes involved in making these spreads and bulk cheese seem to be organized to deliver the least benefit in the greatest bulk. Examine a package of these processed cheeses and notice one interesting thing: by law, and thank the

Pure Foods and Drugs Act for that, they are required to state that most of these cheeses are from forty to fifty percent water. Of course they call water by a more refined name: moisture. So, to begin with, you are being cheated of half of your food dollar when you buy processed cheese,, If you need any further warning before you strip your kitchen of these three food frauds, then let me supply it at once.

White sugar causes tooth decay. It cuts the appetite to the point where more valuable foods are eliminated from your menu, thus robbing you of your natural heritage of a good balanced diet.

White flour and white bread fill you with the least useful portion of the wheat, since the germ of the wheat is removed in the production of such flour. In addition, baked goods made of white flour are filled with various chemicals to whiten and preserve them. None of these are guaranteed to preserve you, however. One such chemical, bromine, has in fact proven to induce insanity in dogs. Certainly bromine will not help the mentality of the average human being one bit. Fortunately, flour millers have been forced by law to discontinue the use of bromine in their processing of flour. The other artificial bleaches and preservatives remain. Avoid them at the penalty of decay and possible insanity or death!

The elimination of these three, white flour, refined sugar and processed cheese, is the beginning of the cleansing process that must be begun on the first: day of your new life. Before we have finished with your kitchen, there is much more to be done. It has often been said that many men dig their graves with a spoon. It can be said further, that many newspaper shopping lists are in fact obituary pages, for the nutritionless foods on their lists starve our bodies into early death. Learn to choose your foods correctly, with an eye to health, not creamy, richly decorated beauty. The rich desserts and sweets that too many of us befoul our stomachs with can best be called "beautiful poisons." It is a fitting phrase.

Learn your food requirements and know the value of every food you eat. You would not put sand in the gas tank of your car. Then why do the same to your body? In chapter 10, I have detailed the exact values involved in each and every food we consume. In the final pages of this book, devoted to diet, I have detailed a splendid diet for eliminatory purposes. I call it the "Return-to-Nature Diet." Begin your life with an *internal bath* and you will soon know what true health can be.

Repairing the injured organs and tissues of your body is not a simple process. Most of us have spent the years of our lives in destroying the magnificent machinery with which we entered this world. "Most men make use of the first part of their life to render the other part wretched." (La Bruyere). You cannot hope to overcome the destruction of years of living out of harmony with nature in any short period of time. You are fortunate in that the equipment of your birth is able to absorb so many shocks, distortions and attacks without collapsing completely under the strain. You cannot expect to repair years of constant abrasion, corrosion and abuse in a matter of days.

The course needed for the repair of your body depends largely upon its condition. There are no two fingerprints alike, and there are no two bodies quite alike. The application of natural methods will depend upon the general health of your body. You may be able to benefit most from one degree of exercise and exertion, others from another. You may respond best to water bathing, others more readily to air and sun.

Grow to understand your body and its characteristics. Know the skin of your entire body as well as you know that of your face. Be conscious of such things as bowel movement, liquid intake, normal temperature and pulse, sleeping habits, etc. These, even pulse and temperature, vary with the individual.

Therefore, become acquainted with your individual body functions and routine. For only by knowing the normal routine of your system can you recognize those deviations from the norm that indicate malfunctions of your body. These changes may not be dangerous in themselves, but they can prepare you for what lies ahead. For they are nature's warnings!

To assist the reader, I have detailed within this book many case histories of those who have combatted decay and disease by natural methods. It is my hope and firm belief that these experiences will prove more than helpful to you.

The maintenance of good health is indeed the simplest of all the tasks that lie ahead of you. Once your body has been cleansed of waste matter and their resultant poisons and the decay of those toxins has been repaired, maintaining good health becomes a simple matter of living the sensible, balanced, natural existence we were all meant to conduct. Natural living, the prevention of disease and decay, is pleasant, uncomplicated and filled with the zest of joyful experience. One month of living in harmony with nature will make pale beside it all those years of complication, frustration and the kind of competitive existence that turns life into a short, worried path from cradle to grave.

Natural living is no great secret that lies hidden within the maze of laboratory equipment and scientific formula, although it is a secret to most of us today. To live in harmony with nature is to observe the laws which early man knew as the only way of life. To sleep well. To eat intelligently. To expose body and soul to the warm, deep and satisfying therapy of sun, water and air.

Why do you suppose it is that these three fundamentals of health, Clean, Repair, Maintain, have so long been ignored? Why is it that even to this day, so many turn to the test tube and the knife for a quick road to health, though often neither of these prove more than immediate means of relief? Why do you suppose it is that even at this late date in history, our men of science continue to be baffled by such seemingly simple conditions as the common cold, fatigue, headaches and rheumatic pains? For the answer to this we will turn in the next chapter to the basis of modern medicine, that sacred cow, the germ theory of disease.

This, then, is my recommendation for the first day of your life. Complete the reading of this book up to and including chapters four and five, dealing with internal and external cleanliness. Study the eliminatory diet. Then prepare for tomorrow. Starting with your first waking moment, begin to live your new life. Prepare for health, happiness and long years of rewarding existence. It can be yours!

III FOUR WAYS TO CONTACT NATURE

"Dust thou art, To
dust returneth"

Modern science prides itself on the manner in which it has been able to extend the lifespan of man. Statisticians point to the fact that, in the western world at least, the living years of modern men have been extended about fifteen years over that of 19th century men. And, though they have no accurate figures to prove these claims, they also assert that in our century, men live more than twenty-five years past the span of life in the middle ages.

Yet, for all purposes, the years referred to, even as far back as the sixteenth and seventeenth centuries, are all drawn from what can be called modern times. The division between modern and ancient civilizations can most accurately be made by drawing a line between that time when men lived upon the land, each growing his own food, each toiling in his own fields, and that moment when huge, dirty, sunless cities of commerce sprang up, tearing men from the soil, removing them from that source of health and natural power which we call mother earth.

Of what importance is this to you in your quest for a sound body, a healthy mental outlook and a long and productive life? Why should you concern yourself with the living habits of men who lived a thousand or even five thousand years before your time? Here again the answer can be found in those areas of the East and Middle-east, China, India and parts of Russia, where even at this late date men boast of life-spans in excess of one hundred years. These people, without exception, live upon the soil. They use the methods of planting, cultivation and harvesting used by man two thousand years ago. They walk barefoot, sleep upon the ground and bathe in running streams. These people live as close to the natural sources of life as men did at the birth of civilization, and resultantly they outlive the town and city dwellers by over seventy years! What are the sources of their natural health? They are four — Earth, Sun, Air and Water!

Once you understand the healing qualities of these four, Earth, Sun, Air and Water, you will be prepared, with the help of these natural agents, to live within the bosom of nature and enjoy her loving care. For nature has provided well for her children. She has created the means of preserving health, happiness and long life and placed them all around you. There is little for you to do beyond recognizing them and applying these natural healers to your own life.

EARTH:

The giant Hercules, according to Greek lore, was ordered to take the golden apples from Antaeus, son of Geea, the earth goddess. Hercules and Antaeus were locked in terrifying combat and it appeared that Hercules would be destroyed, until he discovered that Antaeus weakened only when he was separated from earth contact, and regaining that contact, he was refreshed and revitalized. Thus Hercules lifted Antaeus into the air and, holding him aloft, was able to strangle the weakened giant.

Myth? Certainly. But what was the origin of this tale? Obviously the early Greeks, descendants of still earlier man, were attempting to record early man's knowledge of the powers that lie within earth itself.

Man, the most complex and highly developed form of life on earth, is yet a product of earth. He feeds upon plant life, which *is* of the soil, and even gains, through plant life, direct elements of the soil such as iron, calcium, phosphorous, chlorine, sodium, and others adding to some twenty-seven in number. When we realize how much of the human body can be identified among the elements found within the earth, we understand how accurate is the biblical adage, "dust thou art."

Adolf Just, one of the greatest names in natural therapy, realized the curative powers of earth more than fifty years ago when he wrote, "Animals and man are as much products of the earth as the plants; in consequence of their higher development, the former have separated themselves from the earth, have become walking nerve-plants. But animals and man are still as much subject to the laws of nature as plants, they still draw their strength and vitality from the earth."

Have you ever slept on the earth, with only the stars for your ceiling? Have you ever thrown yourself upon the thick green carpet of earth and permitted your body to become one with sun and soil? Have you ever walked barefoot through grass, sand or rich farm soil and felt the glorious glow of earth and green move slowly up from your feet with a warm, healing sensation that soon swelled throughout your body? If so, then you have directly experienced the power which has been called earth-magnetism. This direct contact of body tissue with the source of all power, earth, produces within men a sense of soothing security, of warm and healing contact such as you have never known before. Children, who have the natural desire to walk barefoot and as bare of clothing as their parents will allow, do not derive their attitudes from involved thought processes. A child is more instinct than intellect. What he wants is what he *feels* he should have. It is only the adult who teaches him the do's and don's of so-called civilization.

There is a natural tendency among us all, at one time or another in life, to get as close to mother earth as we possibly can. And, once doing so, we find the kind of satisfaction and feeling of true well-being that we have never before known. Is this just a mental attitude? Are we all deluding ourselves? No! This is no figment of all our imaginations. It is a real and important factor in the health of mankind, this earth-magnetism.

For example, outdoor sleeping was never required of the patients at Yungborn, but facilities were provided for those who found comfort in it. In a beautifully wooded area of the estate, simple shelters, open on ail four sides, were constructed. These shelters which we called "air-houses" were equipped with cots for those who preferred to sleep out of doors but were not convinced of the value of direct earth-contact. Others, of course, rejected the beds completely and slept on the bare ground of these shelters. Still others preferred to remain indoors at night.

It was interesting to me to see many visitors at Yungborn pass from indoor to outdoor sleeping and, in some cases, even to actual earth sleeping. One such patient is recalled to my mind immediately. H. B. was a wealthy New York man of about fifty who possessed most of those things which are supposed to insure health and happiness. He had a flourishing business, a wholesome family life, a helpful and intelligent wife and all the creature comforts which his wealth could purchase. But despite this, H. B. was one of the most nervous and unhappy souls I have ever met.

For a period of three years, this man's family physician had attempted various treatments for the insomnia that was the bane of H. B.'s life. A nerve specialist and a famed psychiatrist had been consulted in the hope that they might have some clue to the patient's sleeplessness. Finally, in desperation, the family doctor recommended a stay at Yungborn.,

In his first week at Yungborn, H. B. totally rejected the idea of sleeping out. He was convinced that lying upon the "hard" ground, without springs or mattresses, would only add to his sleeplessness. Indeed, he called it a "crackpot idea". By the end of that week, an eliminatory diet and frequent air and sunbaths had brought a marked improvement to his general condition, but the insomnia continued without let-up.

H. B. was early to recognize the general improvement that Yungborn treatment had brought his nerve-wracked body. Thus it was that in the second week, with a rather adventurous attitude, he joined some of those who practiced outdoor sleeping. For three nights he slept on a cot in one of the shelters. The immediate change was noticeable, even astounding He went about the sanitorium grounds each morning, reporting to anyone who would listen that he had just had his first decent night's sleep in three years.

There is a post script to this story. It is in a letter which was received at the sanitorium about two months after a new and thoroughly revitalized H. B. bid us goodbye. I quote from it briefly, not as proof of the benefits of earth-contact, but because of the interesting suggestion he offered:

"Looking backward, it is amusing for me to realize that less than twelve weeks ago I was the fellow who looked out at those outdoor sleepers and said 'a bunch of crackpots!' For here I am, just a short while after, practicing that same wonderful course two or three nights a week. I'll bet you people are wondering how a city dweller like me is able to get a couple of good nights outdoor sleep each week without being tagged the neighborhood 'nut'. Well, it was simple enough. The day I drove back to town from Yungborn, I spotted a small lot of ground for sale just a few miles in from the Hudson River on the New Jersey side. I made a note of the owner's name and contacted him as soon as I got back to town.

"Before the week was out I owned that quarter acre of New Jersey. And inside of two weeks of weekend labor, I had one of those air-houses that you people use at Yungborn, all my own. Just a simple little shelter, open on all sides and provided with plenty of hot and cold running breezes from the river. And this is the part that will tickle you — I built it myself."

The rest of the letter was a glowing testimonial to natural therapy. But I have quoted from it really to indicate how a little imagination and determination can bring even the city dweller closer to the real power of health and happiness. While H. B. could have afforded many times the expense involved in building his little shelter, he could never have bought the joy of creation that he obtained by hammering it together himself. Even at present prices, such an air-house can be built for less than the cost of a week's stay at some country resort. And the life-long pleasure that your own sun and air-house will provide can never be counted in dollars and cents.

Outdoor sleeping is believed by many to be the finest form of earth-contact obtainable. But this is certainly not the only means of deriving the benefits of the soil from which we all spring. Two other practices, which are even more commonly used than outdoor sleeping, are readily obtainable to all. The first of these being the most primitive and traditional form of earth-contact, that of walking barefoot upon the soil.

The power which we speak of as earth-magnetism has been likened to other forms of natural power. The comparison between earth-magnetism and electricity, for example, is a rather logical one. The earth itself can be compared with an electromagnet. Indeed many physicists, chief among them Dr. Albert Einstein, have proven that it is this very force of magnetism which holds the earth and all other plants within their orbits, or space-paths. Naturists contend that this amazing force of which Einstein speaks is, in fact, earth-magnetism.

If you conceive of earth-magnetism as a force similar to electricity and having similar properties, then you can see why contact between the earth and any one area of the body is as effective as the full contact that takes place when you lie outstretched upon the ground. If you want to send a charge of electricity through a mile of wire, it is not necessary for you to place the entire length of wire in contact with the source of electricity. By placing just one end of the body in contact with earth-magnetism, we are able to supply the entire body with the benefits derived therefrom.

The parallel between earth-magnetism and electricity becomes even more interesting when you realize the effect that water has upon both. Everyone should by now be aware that water creates excellent electrical contact. For that reason you are warned never to go swimming during an electrical storm and never, under any circumstances, to answer the telephone or switch on an electrical appliance when your hands or feet are wet. The relationship between water and electricity is well known to you. But are you aware that this property of water also applies to earth-magnetism? For many years now, nature-wise folks have practiced walking barefoot upon dewy grass. Those who have felt the health benefits of earth magnetism know that early morning or evening dew upon the grass increases the degree of contact between earth and body. And, for most of us, such walks are a far easier and more practical means of receiving the benefits of earth-magnetism than by outdoor sleeping.

One further means of receiving the blessing of earth contact demands your attention. Father Kneipp, the pioneer in water-therapy, was among the first to advocate walking in running streams. The cool, crystal clear water that swirls about your legs as you walk through the soft silt or on the rocks of a running stream has been credited with the most fabulous effects upon rheumatic and circulatory conditions of all sorts. In the absence of any other means, wading in your own bath tub with the water gushing full force will also be a benefit. In the annals of drugless medicine, you will find countless reports of near-crippled patients who have had torturous pain washed from their limbs by such walks through wet grass or fresh running streams.

These are the three principal sources of earth-contact which are available to you: outdoor sleeping, barefoot walks and water treading. No matter where you live, one of these is accessible. At first you may find it difficult integrating a daily contact with God's good earth into your existence. But if you are determined to know the glories of real health and happiness, you will find a way. I cannot urge you too strongly to find some way to begin your practice of earth-contact at once.

I would like to see the day, and it may not be too far off, when every family, city-bred or not, will own a piece of land upon which it can live in the manner which nature had intended for us all. For only on earth, with the sun, fresh water and clean air of the open country, can we expect to find the true source of health, the harmony with nature that spells long and vital life for us all.

SUN:

Let me begin with a warning: a little knowledge is a danger-ous thing. "Within the past twenty years, sun bathing has be-come a popular movement and it is certainly about time. But, unfortunately, with this discovery of the powers and benefits of the sun, has not come a full knowledge and sane approach to sun bathing. Many advocates and practitioners of sun bathing seem to think they have found some cure-all. They are not aware that nature offers no single cure-all. Only the constant practice of living in harmony with all the laws of nature can be considered the natural cure-all. No one law of nature can be practiced successfully apart from all else. Use earth and sunlight and you will never want for the miracles of nature. Notice as the sun moves through the sky, how plant leaves turn to it, anxious to absorb every moment of sun's rays available to them.

But here is my warning. The sun, while it is a wonderful source of energy and health, is also a dangerous and harmful force when not dealt with intelligently. Over-exposure to the sun can lead to painful, even fatal burns, skin-cracks, bleeding, headaches, dizziness, and nervous disorders. You have your choice, you may take your sun in intelligent measures, day by day, with resultant health. Or you may go about it haphazardly, skipping it for days in a row and then attempting to make it up by taking long periods, hours on end, of harmful sunlight. Again, the choice is yours.

The intelligent person will, of course, introduce himself to the sun in a gentle manner, taking no more than ten minutes of total exposure on the first day, and lengthening this period until twenty or thirty minutes of exposure are reached. No more than half an hour of sunlight at any one time is capable of being absorbed and used by the body. Keep that in mind. A suntan is actually nature's safety device, which filters the harmful rays of too much sun. Also keep in mind that the skin oils of your body help you to derive Vitamin D from the sun. Therefore do not wash those oils from the body before sun-bathing. Do not bathe or shower just before your sun treatment.

But most important of all, the sun by itself is not a natural therapy. Man was not meant to lie directly under the rays of the sun. Not merely because such direct exposure can be harmful, but also because the healing qualities of the sun can best be found when combined with the plant life around us.

In Africa, where the people are constantly exposed to sunlight all year around, you will find that they attempt to avoid the direct rays of the sun wherever possible. In the jungle, the sunlight *is* filtered through the trees. And in the African villages, you will find that great sun-breaks of leaves and branches are built along the streets, filtering the sun's rays from direct contact with the body. These "green roofs," in addition to being picturesque, actually recreate the conditions of the jungle, where the sun is also filtered through leaves before touching the body. This seems to have been nature's intention from the start. Not direct and parching exposure, but filtered, cool and enjoyable sunlight which will not concentrate on any one area of the body and harm the tissues therein.

Thus, the natural sun bath should be taken in the semi-shade of trees and brush. This does not mean to avoid the sun entirely. To gain the power of the sun, you must feel its warmth. But this is best done beneath the green, where the rays are filtered and where the process of growth which sun brings to trees and plants can become a part of our sun-bathing. Where the tree-filtered sunlight is not readily available, much the same advantages can be derived from merely covering the body with leaves and grass that have been dampened with fresh water, much as dew dampens growing plants. Once you have felt the wonders of plant-filtered sunbathing, you will never again return to the scorching direct-contact method.

All sunbathing, of course, is best done with as little clothing as possible. This does not mean, however, that nudity is essential or even beneficial. In particular, the sex organs of the body should never be exposed to direct sunlight for any length of time. Much as the exposure of male and female sex organs to X-ray has proven extremely destructive, so such exposure to direct sunlight will induce sterility.

To attain maximum exposure (always remembering to protect the sex organs), it is best to have some means of withdrawing yourself from view. No matter how we may attempt to educate others, there are always those who will fail to understand the total morality of living in harmony with nature. For this, in fact, is the highest morality known to man. If you have a convenient hideaway, a roof or balcony, field, wood or solarium, or even a sun-lit part of your own room, you may enjoy your private sunbath with complete satisfaction. You need a space no more than three feet: wide and six feet long, with just enough room for a relaxing bath of sunlight. Something in that much space is possible for all of us.

AIR:

It is all around us. We walk through it, blow, sniff and swallow air the day through. And like the familiarity that breeds contempt, we think about it possibly a half dozen times during a life. We think of it when swimming under water, the lungs bursting for air. We worry if there will be enough air to support us in tight quarters; if the baby will die for lack of it if the blankets cover its head. City folks marvel at it when they step out into the country and find a new and refreshing substance entering their lungs. And that: is about as much thought as we afford the ever-present air.

Benjamin Franklin, in a letter to a friend, Dr. Dubourg, wrote the following: "You know that cold water as a hardening agent has been very popular here for a longish time, but it seems to me that the shock of cold water is, generally speaking, always too strong. I found it far more agreeable for my own constitution to bathe in another of the elements; I mean, in fresh air. I therefore get up every morning and sit in my room, reading or writing, completely naked, for half an hour to one hour, according to the season. This air-bath is not unpleasant in the least; and when, as often happens, I afterwards creep back into bed, before dressing, I complete my night's rest with a further hour or two of the most beautiful sleep imaginable. I have found no evil effects resulting from the habit, and believe, not only that it in no way harms my health, but on the contrary, contributes to its maintenance. I should therefore like to refer to this air-bath in future as an energizing, strengthening bath."

This early estimate of the health-giving powers of air, by the illustrious Ben Franklin, is, if anything, an understatement. Air is primary not only to life, but to health as well. You are not interested only in remaining alive, but rather in remaining alive in a state of good health. And, I repeat, air *is* one of your major allies in this struggle.

Take a deep down breath that swells your abdomen. Concentrate upon the air intake as it fills your lungs, expands your chest and flexes your diaphragm. Exhale it slowly, evenly, through your lips. Now, so far as most of us are concerned, this is the sole duty of air in the maintenance of life and health, this thing we call breathing. But, if you believe this to be so, you are wrong!

Breathe once more, consciously! Let it out again. That is a complete breath cycle. Yet, while you were completing that two-fold act, air was being "breathed" by a hundred thousand different openings upon the surface of your skin. That is, the pores of your skin were exhaling if you were allowing them to. You cannot breathe with your nose through three layers of cloth. Neither can your skin. In fact, were you to paint your body from head to toe, thus sealing up the pores, you would die within one hour. Every excess layer of clothing you wear is actually suffocating the pores of your skin. "What difference does that make?" you ask.

A man cuts his finger. He washes it out and bandages the wound with cotton and gauze. Each day he changes the bandage, maintaining it for five or six days. At the end of that time, the wound is not completely healed, but the man, disgusted with the bandages that seem to do so little good, throws them away. Two days later, the wound is healed completely. Why?

A city-bred woman, nervous, distraught, plagued by insomnia, rides out into the country only to lose her way at nightfall. Frightened at the thought of driving back to the city, she rents a room from a local farm woman. The room is large, unheated, weather beaten. Wind whistles in through the eaves. "What a horrible place!" she thinks. "No steam heat. Cold air shipping through it. Ugh, I'll never sleep a moment in this place." But the farm woman bundles her off to bed and the night begins. The wind shrieks through the trees. Tree branches scratch at the window. The old house creaks with the burden of its years. And here is this city woman without her ear plugs, no mask to shut out the light of the moon, no consoling radiator to pour its comforting steam into her face, no sleeping pills to drug her senseless. And here she sleeps almost from the moment her head hits the pillow. When she awakens in the morning, she feels more refreshed, more in favor of living, than she can recall having ever been before. Why?

Air! The air you breathe is the "mysterious" medicine that helped heal the man's wound. The air that whistled through that old house is the "sleeping pill" that lulled the city-lady to complete rest and left her feeling alive and thrilled to be so.

Air-bathing, as practiced by Benjamin Franklin, is as old as man. The less clothing man wore (and early man wore little), the more he bathed himself in life-giving air. The more he bandaged his body in cotton, wool and nylon, the more he "protected" it with walls of wood, brick and steel, the less nourishment his body received from the air of our planet. I say our planet, since the atmosphere of other worlds does not contain the mixture of vapors we call air. And these other atmospheres will not support human life.

Peculiarly enough, though men have always known of the importance of air in their lives, they have constantly moved away from the kind of life that would avail them of the curative powers of the air. Of course, we have never strayed so far as to try to live without breathing, although some of the tight starched collars that men once wore, and the steel and bone corsets worn to this day by most women, are a step in the direction of strangulation. Now, try a small and simple experiment. Go to the window, open it wide and stand before it. Hold your breath for as long as you are able. Then breathe deeply and slowly a half-dozen times. Feel the air as it fills your lungs and expands your abdomen. Pull your head way back and let yourself enjoy each deep lungful. Don't wait until you have finished this page or this chapter. Do it now! What you will learn in front of your own window in six deep breaths will teach you more than all the words I know. Do it now!

How was it? Did you hold your breath for half a minute or longer before enjoying the full power of the fresh air? If so, you discovered something you never knew before. Air has its own odor, it *is* not odorless as we thought. You can practically *taste* the wonderful elixir called air. And while you were drinking at one of nature's most important pools, you could feel your whole body filling with a new vibrance, a new vigor.

There is a headiness that comes with deeply breathed air that no champagne, no wine or liquor, can ever create. And all this from six breaths of air.

What do you suppose fifteen minutes of this would do for you each day? And not merely fifteen minutes of nose breathing: what if you were to spend that brief time in body breathing? Ahh, what a glorious morning you have before you. For tomorrow you will have taken your first air-bath!

AIR BATHING:

The proper air bath does not truly begin in the morning. The first step in approaching this wonderful therapy should be taken at night. It is a simple step, for it merely consists of opening your bedroom window. I am aware that few people sleep in a completely closed room, though some foolhardy ones among us still do. But nevertheless, I am going to ask that *all* of you, no matter what your past practice, open the window in your bedroom at least two inches more this evening than you did the night before. The reason that I ask this of all is because experience has shown that about only one person in a thousand permits the proper amount of air to flow through his or her sleeping chamber. Engineers have said that, were it not for the little chicks and crevices around the windows and doors of our houses, the cracks of loose construction, many of us would suffocate to death!

Don't forget, at least two more inches of air space in that window tonight. And this must be a year-round matter, controlled by the seasons. In other words, this summer and in the future, see to it that your window is open two inches more than last summer. This winter make certain you have two inches more of air-space in your window than in the past. Start this practice tonight. This is the beginning of your life-long air bath.

In the morning, when you awake, throw off the covers and remove your night clothes, if you must wear them. Now you are ready for the bath. Begin by stretching your body fully upon the bed. Stretch until you can feel the muscles pull in every direction. Now a couple of big yawns will help you shake off the sleepiness. And follow that with a very simple exercise. Sit up in bed and relax. Let your head hit your chest, so to speak. Now roll your head slowly, in a small circle, around the pivot of your neck and shoulders. Don't tighten your neck muscles to do this, let gravity do half the job for you as your head comes to the top of the arc and rolls naturally back to the base. All these are preliminaries, but how well you feel after them!

Now it's time to move around. The amount of exercise necessary during your air bath depends largely upon the temperature of the room. In the winter you may find it helpful to do a few deep knee bends and ceiling stretches, this circulates your body and warms the outer tissues. In the summer, almost any kind of light exercise will do, even the little things you have to do to prepare your clothes for the day will be sufficient agitation for the air bath. But keep moving! Some men find it convenient to shave during their air bathing period. I know one lovely lady of fifty who combines her air bath with a morning dance. She turns on her record player and begins the morning with soft dance music. That is one of the happiest exercises I can think of. Besides, research during the past ten years has proven the wonderful use that can be made of music, particularly in the early part of the day. A soft melody and some medium rhythm is the best alarm clock.

The need for exercise during the air bath grows out of the bathing process itself. When you lie in a tub of water, you always move about, splashing water here and there to make certain that the entire body is well bathed. And in water bathing, you apply a wash cloth or brush to the surface of the skin by way of assisting the water to flush the top layer of tissue. The same is true in the air bath. Exercise, body motion of any sort, actually washes the body with the flow of purifying air and, like the wash cloth and brush, lends a penetrating action to the air. And so a primary rule in air bathing is, *keep moving!*

The nude body, in motion, accomplishes two tasks: air is fed to the skin surface and the muscles of the body are activated. Nature's laws above all demand motion. Static matter does not long remain alive. If you want your body to live and grow each moment of your life. You must see to it that every area of the body receives daily exercise of one sort or another. The degree of exercise will vary with the condition of the individual. There are good muscle-toning exercises for every age and condition of health.

One further word about your first air bath. A major benefit of air bathing *is* the wonderful stimulus it supplies to the skin. A sallow, pimply and unhealthy looking skin can be brought to a new glow of life through a series of morning or evening air baths. (Though morning baths are preferable, evening baths, even with the sunless night air, are especially useful to those of us who cannot accommodate our daily routine to earlier bathing. What is important is not so much the time of day as the loyalty you demonstrate to these daily air baths.)

The key to maintaining a healthy skin through air bathing lies in the skin rubs and massages that should accompany these daily baths. The skin, like all of our body, needs regular exercise and stimulation. This stimulation will not only improve the condition of the skin itself, but will provide you with a tingling and bubbling sensation that comes with living in tune with nature. Before you have completed your first air bath, try this series of skin attentions and see if you don't come away from it feeling as though you have just sipped long and well from the fountain of youth.

1. During the exercises that accompany the air bath, rub your arms, thighs, abdomen, chest, back and all portions of the body within reach. This should be no patty-cake process, but rather a brisk rubbing motion interspersed with slapping and grasping of the skin.

2. Purchase a good coarse towel or rubbing cloth as soon as possible and finish air each air bath with a brisk dry toweling of the entire body.

3. Never permit the well exercised body, damp with the healthful perspiration of exercise and stimulation, to remain still. Keep moving during the bath, exercise and rub. And, above all, dry yourself well upon the completion of the bath and get into good, warm clothing. Never, under any circumstances, must you allow yourself to become chilled. I know that there are people who seem to believe that the more you punish your body, the more you will strengthen it. This is a dangerous concept. Air bathing will harden the body to the atmosphere and strengthen it against the colds, chills and nasal disturbances common to so many.

But bodily discomfort is not the same thing as hardening or strengthening the body. On the contrary, an uncomfortable body is one which is on its way to disrepair. Nature means for us to live in comfort and ease. Shocking and disturbing our natural comfort is a hindrance, not a help to Nature. Therefore, avoid chilling your body at all cost!

This, then, is your air bath, or at least the beginning of it. For, although the organized air bath is a matter of a few minutes daily, you are involved in the process of air bathing each moment of your life. It is impossible for you to keep the air from reaching some part of your body at every moment, although many people, the over-dressers, certainly give it a good try.

Since the air is constantly bathing the exposed portions of your body, you can help nature in this task simply by wearing the kind of sensible clothing that will permit the maximum of air contact throughout the day.

Stiff collars and tightly knotted ties are out of the question for the sensible man. In the same way, garters, corsets and overly binding brassieres are plain foolishness for the women. Choose your clothes with a view to providing the maximum amount of comfort. Loosely fitted, soft spun materials are best. Women seem to be moving in a good direction these days, with their bare-backed dresses and short skirts. But the designer who introduced slacks to the female sex was doing them a distinct disservice. Unless a woman is involved in the kind of activity that really calls for such attire, I would suggest that slacks be discarded from the female wardrobe.

In a like manner, I would suggest that men give up the practice of wearing long trousers in the summer, when the natural warmth provided by the sun makes them totally unnecessary. Just as I would prefer to see women give up the wearing of stockings as early as the season will permit. I would advise men to wear shorts the moment the weather permits. And, in addition, light summer attire can be worn year-round in a properly-heated apartment or house. Most important of all, never over-dress. The body must constantly be protected against chill. But there is nothing that invites a chilling breeze like a body that has been over-dressed and over-heated.

Spring, summer, fall and during mild winter days you have an excellent opportunity to take your air-bathing outdoors. The first day that the weather permits, the air bather should rise fifteen or twenty minutes earlier than usual, dress lightly and go outdoors after his usual morning regimen, beginning the day with a brisk walk. Where a walk through field or forest is obtainable, the air bath is most fully enjoyable and beneficial. These walks should be enjoyed barelegged and barefooted, or with light sandals of cork or leather (the less that lies between you and earth-contact, the better.) Never, never use rubber composition soled shoes, which insulate you from the benefits of earth contact. The barefoot or barelegged walker will never suffer the rheumatic or circulatory disorders that go with overheating and perspiration of the legs when these are clothed in stockings, socks and trousers.

Some time ago, a middle-aged man, whose initials were A.M., suffered from very painful legs and backaches, and asked for advice. His sales job called for him to be constantly on his feet. I suggested certain water baths, air bathing and, particularly, strengthening the feet through barefoot walks. He rejected the thought of walking barefoot in his yard, since his neighbor, an older man, had a particularly caustic wit that he used to chide others. Asked which he would prefer to eliminate, his aching feet, or his cynical neighbor, A. M. decided to give the barefoot walks a try, but he was obviously concerned about his nagging neighbor.

A month later, I chanced to visit A. M. at his suburban home. He was raking some leaves on the lawn — barefoot. He told me of the wonderful results the baths and walking had brought, results which I could see for myself as he strutted painlessly about the yard. Then he introduced me to a friend across the way who was also working in his yard. I recognized him from A. M/s earlier description as the scoffing neighbor whose jeers had worried my friend. But A. M. obviously no longer needed to fear his neighbor's caustic humor. For, lo and behold, Mr. Cynic was now working barefoot in his own yard. So much for the scoffers!

Now that you have learned the wonders of air bathing, use this knowledge well. It is a major mile along the road to health. Start at once and never let a day pass without your air bath. Begin with short, five minute sessions. Extend the time day by day until you are able to bathe in air for periods of fifteen minutes at a time. No more than fifteen minutes a day will be needed to guarantee the benefits of one of nature's greatest gifts — the air bath!

WATER:

I have left for last the most common! y used bathing agent of all, water. While many have overlooked the healing qualities of earth, air and sun, there is hardly a place on earth where one or another kind of water therapy is unknown.

Water baths of various sorts, sulfur, steam, pressure baths (affusions), etc., have been a part of human healing for thousands of years. And, if you have observed the life of animals, both domestic and wild, you know why it: is safe to presume that the first man upon earth sought out the healing power of water.

If you have heard how the deer or other animal when it is sick or injured, will crawl to the nearest water hole to wallow in the healing power of earth and water, and rise in a short while, returned to health, you must know how basic water therapy is. More meaningful than the water pilgrimage of sick animals are the regular bathing habits of these creatures. Since they lack reasoning powers, it cannot be said that these animals have recognized the adage, "cleanliness is next to Godliness." Not reason, but instinct, drives deer, antelope and cow to the banks of river and lake. In almost every case, the routine of bathing is the same. This procedure is the same among almost all animals excepting man. Here again man has strayed from the path of nature.

The deer and other animals greatly enjoy their regular baths as you can attest, if you have ever suddenly come upon them during their ablutions. And you would have also noticed that these animals never submerge their bodies beyond a point corresponding to the human abdomen. Enjoying the water as they apparently do, still these simple products of nature will never immerse themselves from head to toe as men do.

There is another bathing trait common to these animals and that is the massage. Since they do not have the developed hands of men, they find it necessary and satisfying to massage their bodies by rubbing them upon the thick black mud of the river bed. They will generally choose a shallow area in which to crouch and massage their bodies, standing on their hind legs to apply needed pressure to the bottoms. In the case of birds, where limbs are developed so as to make it possible, they will generally complete their baths by rubbing their bodies with their wings until they are sufficiently dry.

This long ago led me to certain conclusions concerning the water bath. Applying these rules at both the Florida and New Jersey sanitoriums, we were able to prove the validity of these conclusions and the importance of proper water bathing to the maintenance of health, sexual virility and long life.

THE NATURAL BATH:

The natural bath should not be taken in hot water. Rivers and streams, with their constant exchange and flow of water, never become more than tepid on the hottest day of the year. And the natural bath was first performed in moving water. While it is not a simple matter for you to bathe yourself in the open air, as your ancestors once did, it is important that you approximate those conditions as nearly as possible.

The room in which you bathe should not be overheated. If air and water are at the same temperature, you will find neither uncomfortable. Begin by filling your tub with three or four inches of water, no more. When you enter the tub, you will find this to be only sufficient to cover the feet, buttocks and sexual organs. This is as it should be for natural bathing.

It is not necessary to use soap in your bath, though this is permissible. Personally, I find the use of a genuine pine oil water softener in the bath to be beneficial. The use of soap for removing dirt is rarely required where bathing is frequent and brisk rubbing of the entire body takes place, both during and after the bath. Soap will serve to dry the skin and remove those natural oils which assist in deriving Vitamin D from sunlight. Go on using as much soap as you wish. But let me only ask that the habit of soaping the body not be permitted to replace the healthful water massage.

The natural bath differs widely in two respects from your regular bathing habits. Your body was not meant to be totally submerged. No living creatures other than fish and amphibians (beaver, seal, otter, etc.) benefit by water submersion. Therefore, your natural bath uses a minimum of water. However, despite the fact that natural bathing involves the use of less water, the application of water to the body is so organized and directed as to benefit your body in a manner unknown to you before your discovery of natural bathing.,

Swift and frequent dousings of water upon your abdominal region is the second characteristic of the natural bath. By cooling and revitalizing the circulation upon and around the abdomen and the organs of reproduction, you will do much to remove the most common causes of sexual sterility. In the case of the female, such dousings will help to alleviate the blood congestion that frequently occurs in this important area of the body and the soothing effects of cool water are quickly produced.

The daily and brisk application of cool water to this region will also help act as a guard against sterility in the male. The over-heating and stagnating enclosure of tight undergarments and athletic supporters is a contributing factor to the loss of male sexual potency.

Following this, the procedure is repeated until the entire body has been stimulated and cleansed. The length of time spent at your natural bath is not significant and will vary according to personal need.

It is important to remain constantly in motion during the natural bath. Since the water is never hot, the chance of chilling the body exists, unless you warm yourself with stimulating action and continuous rubbing. This rubbing motion should be continued after you have left the tub and until the body is dry. Towels are unnecessary in the natural bath and their use will deprive you of the stimulating effects of the drying rub.

If you have conducted your natural bath properly, you will not be subject to chill and you may even be able to follow it with an air bath. The air bath is most beneficial when it can be used it conjunction with the natural bath which opens the pores of the skin and permits the entire surface of your body direct contact with the healing qualities of air.

Water is possibly the most vital and versatile of all natural agents. Its uses and benefits are varied and many. In addition to the external bath, water is used internally as in the various colonies (enemas) and liquid diets that cleanse the interior of your body as the natural bath cleanses your surface tissues. All of the healthful uses of water will be discussed in succeeding pages. None should be overlooked in the quest for joyous health.

Earth, Sun, Air and Water are four of nature's greatest agents in the creation and maintenance of health and longevity. Each serves an important purpose in the great and glorious scheme of life, health and happiness, called nature's cycle. Live with and apply each to your own existence and your life will be the fuller, richer and longer for it.

IV.   A LIVE FOOD FOR A LIVE LIFE

*"Other men live to eat, while I eat
to live. "*   Socrates

ONE OF the most important areas of natural living is
the study and application of natural nutrition. Food is the fuel of
human life. Food, as Nature supplies it, is the purest source of
the power needed to drive and revitalize your system. It is important for you to realize the two major tasks performed by what
you eat.

1.   Food supplies you with energy. You must provide your
body with sufficient energy to accomplish its daily tasks. This
is fundamental to life— even the poorest and most devitalized
existence.

2.   Food replenishes the dying tissues of your body. The constant motion within your body requires never-ending replace-
ment of tissue. A balanced diet of natural foods will supply all
the vitamins and minerals necessary to replace the lost tissues.
The absence in your diet of even one of the many elements of
nutrition spells waste, damage and decay to some organ of the
body. One sick organ will smash the chain of life within your
system.

We are all on a diet from the first moment of human conception. What the mother feeds upon provides the diet of the

unborn child. The wife and mother does most of the shopping and cooking for the family. Hence, it is she who determines the family diet. That is why it is comforting to see you women of America increasing your interest in nutrition. But this rate of increased interest in the food you eat is still not enough to begin to cope with the enormous problem of malnutrition that imperils the health of our people.

Malnutrition is a common ailment in our country. It is strange to realize that people who live in the wealthiest country in the history of the world suffer so widely from undernourishment. Malnutrition is not alone an economic problem. The wealthiest homes in any city often hold the poorest diet and most under-nourished bodies in the town.

Malnutrition is the silent killer. It lives upon ignorance and flourishes in a climate of complacency. If you refuse to choose your foods with the care and understanding that good nutrition demands, then you have opened your door to every disease and ailment known to man. Colds, headaches, constipation, loss of sight and hearing, fatigue, rheumatics, premature senility, and much more may be directly traced at one time or another to the poverty of nutrition.

The nutritional specialists, as well as "food faddists" must share some of the responsibility for the poor diet habits of the nation. Many of these specialists have only helped to confuse the public still further with a maze of charts, diagrams and secret formulas which demand a dozen college degrees to be understood. Some of these learned men and women seem to feel that the more confusion they create, the more dependent upon their "secret" wisdom the layman will become.

Good nutrition is no secret! It is common sense. Do not let the food faddists and vitamin fanatics confuse you into a state of despair as they did one young woman I met.

Some time ago, while lunching in my diet food shop in New York City, ï found myself in conversation with the charming private secretary to the president of an advertising agency. She was obviously not aware of my work in the field of dietetics nor of my interest in the restaurant in which we both happened to be eating; Since we were lunching in a food shop which specialized in meals prepared with a view toward better health, our conversation very naturally found its way to talk of nutrition.

A co-worker had introduced Carol to our store two months earlier and since that time she had chosen her food from the shop's menu and the diet charts she found in several editions of Nature's Path magazine. She was quick to tell me of the wonderful changes she had noticed in her own health in that short time. No one could fail to notice her wonderful coloring, the bright gleam in her eyes, the beautiful form of her well fed body.

During the recent wonderful months, while Carol had been reconditioning her body and appetite, one problem kept presenting itself. She explained that after all that time, she still had to carry the vitamin-calorie booklet with her wherever she went to assist her in choosing food. She complained that the food charts with the letters and numbers and strange words — Vitamin A, B complex, Vitamin C, niacin, riboflavin, etc., etc., — all of these were confusing to her. She understood them while she read them from the booklet, but they never stayed in her head. I had to agree with her. I explained that these words and code letters had been created by nutritionists and bio-chemists, specialists in the field of food research. They had created this code, so to speak, to help them in simplifying their work — one letter or word stood for whole series of qualities.

Take Vitamin A, for instance. The A vitamin, first discovered, is an important food factor in the preservation of healthy mucous linings, nose, throat, eyes, etc. Vitamin A is also the little fellow who helps your hair to grow and assists in keeping your skin smooth and unmarked, though this is his secondary job. Lately, we've come to realize how important Vitamin A is in preventing such eye disorders as night blindness. Now you see, it took me a whole paragraph to explain what Vitamin A does. That is the chief reason why code letters and numbers were chosen for some of our food values. By saying; "Vitamin A" you immediately describe all of these things to the person who deals with nutrients every day of the year. But what about the average person, the housewife, worker and businessman?

Carol started me thinking about all of this, and I began to realize how important it is for us to develop a parallel system for recalling the special values contained in each food. What was needed was some simple way of identifying the life-giving properties in our food. That lead me to the realization that each of the vitamins and minerals and others could be named after the particular job it best accomplishes.

Vitamin A, as we said, helps protect our nose and throat against infection, our eyes against strain and blurred vision. Now while it is true that Vitamin A is also effective in preserving healthy hair and skin, its major job seems to be **the** protection of our eyes, nose and throat. Then, while continuing to designate this valuable food factor by its proper name, Vitamin A, why not construct a second name which would identify the health-giving properties of Vitamin A? I did just that. So from here on through this book, you will notice that I refer to "Vitamin A Foods" as well as "Eye, Nose and Throat Foods."

Vitamin B Complex: This wonderful group of life-givers tends to stay together in one happy family. Thus, where one member of the Vitamin B Complex is found, you will usually find the others close behind. This group breaks down into three major units, Vitamin B-1 or Thiamin Vitamin B-2 or Riboflavin, and last, but not least, Niacin.

Vitamin B-1 (Thiamin) aids appetite, growth, fertility, supplies you with energy and soothes your nerves. Since its most valuable contribution is maintaining your nerve tissues in a state of good health, in the future we will refer to all foods rich in Thiamin as B-1 foods or "Nerve Foods."

Vitamin B-2 (Riboflavin) helps provide a healthy complexion, avoid ariboflavinosis, protect your lips and mouth against infection and strengthen your eyesight. Following the rule that calls for naming these food factors for the *major* task they perform, we will now speak not only of Vitamin B-2, but of the "Clear Complexion" vitamin as well.

Niacin is that part of the B-complex which protects you against pellagra, a nasty skin and nerve disorder. Niacin also aids in digestion and helps you to fight fatigue and avoid diarrhea. Like its brothers, B-1 and B-2, Niacin protects your oral (mouth) and mental health. In past years, when the nation's diet was even less balanced than today, pellagra was a common disease, particularly in the South. Today, with pellagra less a danger to skin and mind, we look more and more toward Niacin to tone up our appetites and aid our digestion to better enjoy all foods. For that reason, I refer not only to Niacin, but to "Good Digestion Foods" as well whenever I speak of foods rich in this vital factor.

Vitamin C; Here is another wonderful vitamin that assists you in defeating bodily infections. The C Vitamin is also required to maintain healthy teeth and gums, fights fatigue and the pains that tend to settle in the joints, and promote healing in wounds and bone fractures. From here on, we will frequently call Vitamin C the "Infection-Fighter."

Vitamin D: The D Vitamin is vital in the proper formation of bones and teeth, prevents rickets, and continues to assist you in maintaining and repairing the skeletal system throughout. Let us begin calling Vitamin D foods, "Bone Builders," as well.

Calcium: This offers help in protecting your skeletal system. Calcium should be remembered most of all for the care it takes of your teeth. Enough calcium each, day would help put every dentist out of business. Calcium does no small job in strengthening the heart and nervous system. So be on the look-out for calcium and we can now also call it our "Dental Friend."

Iron and Copper: These two metals, small deposits of which are found in many foods, particularly leafy green vegetables, insure your blood supply against anemia. This strengthening of the blood supply helps combat common fatigue and year round Spring Sickness. Considering the job which iron and copper carry out for us, I think they deserve to be sometimes referred to as the "Blood Bank."

Phosphorous: Here is another mineral that you need in your diet. Phosphorous helps to regulate your glandular systems and does its part in shaping a good skeletal system. From now OP we may often speak of phosphorous as the "Gland Regulator."

Iodine: Someone once asked me why he should eat foods containing iodine, when the drinking of iodine was a common means of suicide. Now don't laugh at this poor man, because when you start talking balanced-diet and the good life with your friends and neighbors, you'll find that many of them are just as poorly informed. So instead of laughing at such a person, the thing to do is to very calmly explain the difference between Tincture of Iodine — a deadly poison used to fight infections which the body would throw off without a druggist's assistance if the body were built up to infection-fighting standards, — and the mineral iodine which is found in many foods and particularly sea foods.

Iodine foods must be a part of your everyday diet if you are to avoid goiter, an enlargement of the thyroid gland which results in a lump or swelling at the front or side of the neck. Iodine not only bolsters your thyroid, but it is also known to have a beneficial effect upon certain mental symptoms. But in conformity, with our rule of naming a nutrient for the chief job it accomplishes, let us call Iodine the "Guard-Against-Goiter".

Other vitamins which are worthy of mention, though at present they do not appear as important in the maintenance of health, are listed below:

Vitamin E: Sometimes referred to as the anti-sterility and anti-abortion vitamin because experiments with various animals indicate that the absence of Vitamin E promotes miscarriage, and sterility in both male and female. Vitamin E is also believed to protect the muscles of the heart and has been used successfully against certain heart diseases.

Vitamins B-6 and B-12: The exact functions of these as yet is uncertain. There are indications that both promote growth, particularly in children, and B-12 is apparently useful in defeating certain form of anemia.

Vitamin P and Rutin: These two are quite similar, and seem to be involved in the important task of building and maintaining healthy blood vessels.

Pab: (Para-Aminobenzoic Acid) Has been used in treatment of typhus and Rocky Mountain Spotted Fever. Proved useful in avoiding gray hair in certain animals, and a growth factor.

I believe that this new method of identifying the various vitamins and minerals in our food supply can be very helpful to us all. I am particularly thankful to that young woman who lunched beside me one day for putting me on the track of a job that needed doing. To Carol and the millions like her, who may have found themselves a bit confused by the many technical terms and codes involved in the language of nutrition experts, I dedicate the above table.

Nutrition is not a very complicated matter, and must not be reserved for specialists. Nature's ways are magnificent in conception and construction, but, at the same time, almost always very simple. Never make the mistake of referring to Nature as some great mystery. For if it is a mystery, then it is one to which every one of us has the key. The key to nature is within you yourself. Look there for it and you will never be disappointed.

Now that we have reached a clearer understanding of food values, let us go on to examine some of the more common foods which, when taken in a balanced diet, will supply you with every nutrient necessary to a longer, healthier life.

In chapter fifteen, you will find a general table of food values with a view to accomplishing four important things*.

1.   To reveal the major values within each food.

2.   To indicate the healing and life-giving qualities of many of these foods.

3.   To inform you as to the best methods for preparing these foods both to preserve the values and to make these foods appetizing.

4.   A handy guide for menu making.

Turn to it now, and begin to study it. This is your guide to healthful eating.

You will notice that I stress the need for appetizing foods and menus. This is extremely important. Food must be appetizing not alone to make life more pleasant, but actually to make your life a healthier and longer one.

Some people, upon first learning the great secrets of health hidden within their diet, set about constructing a food plan to extend and improve their lives without giving a single thought to the flavor and look of the food they eat. They have forgotten a simple fact: the person who eats his food without interest or pleasure does not receive all the food values he should from that food. Why? Simply because the mental attitude you bring to the table effects your digestive system.

Appetizing food causes the digestive juices to flow upon the sight and scent of it. The jump of digestion begins the moment you see and sniff the food you are about to eat. If those juices are stimulated by a handsome, pleasant smelling and tasty dish, then they will soften each bite of food before it reaches the lower digestive tract and make the job of the stomach that much easier.

Food that is unappetizing, carelessly prepared, is swallowed in hard and indigestible lumps. It is difficult, at best, for the stomach to digest a meal, of that sort. The result? Indigestion, for one, constipation, for another, and a loss of much of the food value. When food is not properly digested, it passes through the body without leaving its full values behind. It is what might be termed "half burned fuel."

The person who eats unappetizing food, chosen for the mineral and vitamin content, should not be too surprised if he or she does not receive the full value of that food and in the end, is prone to colds, sore throats, headaches, fatigue and much more. His food is being wasted simply because he refuses to interest himself in the pleasure of food. *The pleasure of foody* that is another important term.

Even including the hasty breakfasts and bread-backed lunches which too many of us rush through, the average person spends about thirty-five days each year just eating. On the basis of what is today considered a normal life span, you use no less than six years of your life in the process of eating! Six years of nothing but eating!

If you knew you would be spending six years of your valuable life with a certain group of people, you would want to be certain that these people were not only intelligent, but also filled with the zest of life that would make those six years truly enjoyable, wouldn't you? The man or woman who sits down to a plate of dishwater (healthful dishwater, of course) and a dry-as-dust salad, has chosen to spend his life with the most boring group of companions imaginable. What a sin against the joy of living. "What a waste of God's greatest creation!

If you are guilty of this sinful waste, then examine your bill-of-fare right now! Change your table companions, not the ones with whom you eat but the tasteless things you have been eating!

I would be very happy indeed, if I could merely indicate what foods will best promote health and extend your life span, and if you could obtain those foods inexpensively and with little trouble. But unfortunately, this is not the case. Is it because the foods commonly grown on our farms are not the correct variety to promote health and sustain life? Not: at all. It is not the kinds of food that are important so much as it is the qualities contained within them. "While asparagus supplies us with Vitamin A, one stalk may supply us with twice as much of this EYE, NOSE AND THROAT aid as another. And it is impossible to tell, merely on sight, just which plant will supply you with the most of any given vitamin or mineral.

It is possible for a head of lettuce to look fresh, crisp, green and as plump as a melon, and for that lettuce to be almost empty of life-giving food values. Why is this so, and what can we do about it? For the answer to this, we must know more about how food is grown, which is explained in our next chapter.

V.   THE FOOD PACKERS ARE STARVING YOU

*"Ashes to
ashes, Dust to
dust."*

WHEN MEN lived upon the land and based their diets on food grown naturally, in the manner intended by nature, they were not faced with the problems and confusion of modern nutrition. Only when they moved from the farms into the cities and ceased to grow their own food supplies from soil which they themselves tended, did they face the dangers of devitalized foods and static diets. For it was then that the food packers, with their mass production and distribution, stepped into the scene.

The food packers were faced with the problem of growing and supplying large populations with food, and doing this at a profit. To sell their food, they made a great effort at "prettifying" it, appealing to the eye, rather than the stomach. They would add bicarbonate of soda to green vegetables to heighten the color. They dyed oranges and grapefruits to give them that ripened look. Preservatives were doused upon jams and jellies, breads and cookies, meats and cheeses, to halt spoilage in transit and storage. The bicarbonate added nothing but color to the vegetables and stole much of the vitamin value. The yellow and orange dyes did not better the green, unripened fruits. And, while the preservatives helped to avoid spoilage, they also, as in the case of white bread, contributed to poisoning your body and destroying your mind.

Possibly the best authority on the subject of food adulteration and poisoning is the United States Government. Here are but a few brief quotes from a congressional committee appointed to investigate the use of chemicals in foods and cosmetics.

"NITROGEN TRICHLORIDE...employed for approximately thirty years in the flour milling industry... In 1946, an English Investigator discovered that dogs fed bread baked from flour treated with nitrogen trichloride developed canine hysteria, commonly referred to as running fits."

"PARA-PHENETYL UREA is a sweetening agent which was used for over 50 years as a sugar substitute for diabetics and others. Until a chronic toxicity study of this substance (was undertaken) several years ago, no investigation of its possible toxic effects when taken in small amounts over an extended period of time, had ever been made. Results of the experiment revealed that para-phenetyl urea is poisonous under such conditions. One firm continued to use it in its food products even after being warned of its toxicity."

"MINERAL OIL has long been regarded as harmless. It had been used in a variety of special dietary foods, particularly salad dressing, as a substitute for food oils. Between 1941 and 1945, evidence became available which showed that mineral oil, when taken with foods, interfered with the absorption of various vitamins. As a result of this evidence, mineral oil is no longer permitted as a food ingredient."

This particular report goes on to list many other chemical agents contained in processed and packaged foods which are detrimental to human health. Emulsifiers, for instance, chemicals used by bakeries to give bread that "more tender" feeling and thus trick the public into believing this baked food to be fresher than it actually is, were found to dilute the nutritive value of foods and present the possibility of actual poisoning. The American Medical Association took the position that so long as these emulsifiers cannot be proven to be harmless, they should not be used in any foods.

Why did such a horrifying condition exist?

The food packers were more interested in maintaining the color, odor and texture that would sell their products than they were in preserving the food values. That is why it became necessary for you to know the contents of every package and can of food you purchased. If the food packers were not interested in protecting you against malnutrition, then you had to do the job yourself.

The greatest sin committed by the large food packers of the nation in their endless attempts to produce bigger and more colorful looking foods is their complete indifference to the conditions of the soil from which our food is produced.

More recently, the packers have shown an increased interest in nutrition. Large research institutes have been endowed by the packers for purposes of analyzing and grading food products. The earlier philosophy of eye-appeal over food value still exists too widely for you to be able to purchase food indiscriminately. Nonetheless, the earlier philosophy of eye-appeal over food value still exists too widely for you to be able to purchase food indiscriminately.

VI NO MATTER WHAT AILS YOU

*"For all the happiness mankind can gain Is
not in pleasure, but in rest from pain."*
— *Dryden*

You HAVE a human body. You own the greatest assemblage of tools, machines, computers and analyzers ever devised. You were complete at birth and you have added nothing since that moment, only developed that which already existed. At birth you were perfection! What are you today?

In the first fifteen to twenty years of life, you existed upon the wisdom and indulgence of others. If others did not eat wisely, you were fed upon their ignorance. If others chose a path that led away from the natural source of health, you were forced to stray with them. Even when you reached that point in life when you fed, clothed and guided your own destiny, your choices had largely been formed by the habits of those who came before you. Each time you learned something new and important in living, you were forced to choose between the lessons taught to you by parent and teacher, and the knowledge that came to you through your own experience. If your life resembles that which most people lead, each such choice has been a difficult one for you.

The errors of the past have played havoc with most of us. Is it any wonder that what was perfection at birth is no longer perfection?

In seeking the path that will return them to the wholesome conditions of their birth, rational-livers have rediscovered the laws of nature. "With this rediscovery, they have returned their bodies to the simple life that brings with it power of health and the glory of long life. By returning their bodies to the most sympathetic climate, the climate provided by earth, sun, water, air. life-foods (those naturally grown and consumed in the state closest to their raw goodness), the rational-livers have found that for which emperors, kings and explorers searched the world over. They have found this, not half-way around the world, but right within themselves and in the earth around them. When you find it, you will have discovered Nature's fountain, of youth.

In the past one hundred years, great discoveries in the field of natural living have been made. These were truly rediscoveries of past life. It is not unusual for valuable information to have been lost to mankind through years of emptiness and ignorance. The steam engine was invented by the Egyptians two thousand years before James Watt rediscovered it and gave this power to the world. The Pharaos of Egypt had no use for steam power when the arms and backs of slaves were so cheap. And so steam power was lost to the world for two thousand years, until industry found use for it.

There have been times in history, too many, when human life was not highly valued. Such is not the case today, and for this we must be thankful. The rediscovery of natural living and the road to true health and long life couldn't come until men valued their own lives for what they were, the greatest conception of the universe.

The fact that thousands of years have intervened between early man with his natural life and present man with his modern and unnatural existence, accounts for the lack of knowledge concerning natural living. There are no documents written by the first men and women to tell us of how they lived in harmony with their natural environment. We are forced, therefore, to learn these things for ourselves.

Natural learning derives, as you would suspect, from the observation of nature. We learned of the natural bath from watching the bathing habits of animals which have not lost their sense of harmony with nature. In the same way, we learned much about dieting, sleeping habits, air and sun bathing and many other matters. Man is not just another animal. He is a highly specialized breed with great powers not found anywhere else in life. Therefore, men cannot expect to live and prosper quite as any other living thing does.

The only other major source of natural knowledge is the human being himself. We watch men and women around us. See how they live. See how they eat, work, sleep and perform the thousand and one daily habits that compose their lives. We draw certain conclusions from these observations and hope that we have found truth. But the area for error is wide.

In knowledge, as in much else, there is safety only in numbers. We can only be sure we have established fact when we have seen it work in enough cases and under the variety of conditions that will convince the disbeliever as well as those ready to be shown. This is the only kind of knowledge I am willing to deal with. Your life is too precious to convert it into a guinea pig for any fad or whim that may come your way.

In this chapter, I have detailed case histories of many common ailments. Though each case history is accurate and refers to one specific individual who found relief from pain and decay through natural therapy, each is also representative of many other such cases. That is to say that space and time will not permit me to illustrate more than one case history for each of these conditions, but the particular case discussed is representative of dozens like it, with the same symptoms and similar therapy applied.

I have used, as source material for these cases, only the histories drawn from the files of our Florida and New Jersey sanitoria. I prefer not to refer to similar cases and courses of therapy outlined in any other book, pamphlet or paper, since I cannot vouch for the conditions or the degree of help brought to the patient by the treatment discussed. I will set down only those things which I myself have witnessed.

As we have already seen, Nature provides us with certain basic natural agents such as earth, air, sun and water, for gaining and maintaining health and longevity. It is important for us to understand these fundamentals well, for they are the foundation of natural living. In the field of natural therapy, there are also basic agents with which we must become well acquainted, since they are fundamental to the treatment of decay and disease. Again and again, you will find these basic natural courses referred to in the case histories outlined. For that reason, it is best that you be introduced to them at once, so that you may better understand their uses and great healing values.

PACKS: Primary in the treatment of many ailments, particularly those involving swollen or sensitive skin tissue, is the pack. There are many forms of packs, each with a special job to accomplish in returning your body to full health. These packs differ in size and temperature and in materials and are referred to as hot, cold, whole, and small, water and clay. When the term pack is applied alone, it is taken to mean a water pack of medium temperature to be applied to the affected area.

At Yungborn, packs were used for two principal functions: to induce stimulation naturally (druglessly) to the blood stream, and to break a fever. When stimulation was urgent the closed pack was used. In breaking a fever, the open pack was always employed. The difference between the two lies in the heavy, dry outer-layer used in the closed pack to deny air to the wet layer and induce perspiration. The open pack can be described as a large compress, exposed to the air where evaporation causes a natural cooling of the body. Extreme caution was always taken, both during the open and closed pack, to prevent the body from being chilled. In the case of fever, the body temperature was constantly measured and the moment that it began to fall, the open pack was removed and the patient wrapped in a light blanket.

Water packs are always applied in a room of comfortable temperature. When used to induce circulation and perspiration (closed packs), care is taken to keep the outer covers dry and the patient comfortably warm. Except when my wife is near by and can check from time to time to be certain that I am well covered, I never remain in the pack overnight. Instead, I withdraw from the pack after thirty to forty-five minutes and dry myself thoroughly, changing the bedclothes if they have become dampened, and then return to a warm, dry bed.

The wet layer of the water pack is made of cotton, linen or other plant cloth (wool and synthetic cloths are not recommended.) The dry outer layer of the pack may be of wool or any other absorbent material. When it is applied to the chest, neck or face, a drop or two of pine scent or cologne may be sprinkled upon it to lend it a pleasant odor.

You must never forget the need to consider mind and body as one and to please both whenever treating one or the other.

A full pack is worn from neck to knees. A terry-cloth bathrobe soaked and wrung out is my favorite material for the full pack, since it is so easy to don. The small pack is of a size suited to the specific area of distress (leg, arm, hip, etc). "Where the pack is to be worn overnight or for an extended period of time, it should be covered with two layers of dry cloth and tied securely in place, without hindering proper blood circulation.

CLAY PACKS: The use of earth in the healing of wounds and the reduction of swelling is among the oldest devices of natural healing. All of us, at one time or another, have applied earth packs to a swollen area, bee sting, etc. Though our ancestors used clay packs with great success, many today tend to shun such natural treatment out of a fear of "dirtiness." It *is* well to remember that man himself, with his slums and tenements, has produced the dirt of the world. Nature has always provided well for her own decay, using it to replenish life.

Those who reject earth on the grounds of dirtiness might as well remove all food from their lives, since food, animal or vegetable, is all produced from earth. As for the dirt that man produces, any mechanic will tell you that dry earth is an excellent cleanser of grease and grime.

At present, the finest clay for purposes of natural therapy *is* obtained from Europe. This is doubtless because the countries of middle Europe have made the most extensive research and practice of drugless healing. I am certain that the increased interest in natural therapy will bring forth vast deposits of similar clays here in the United States. Clay can be obtained at local health food stores and through central distributors. Where you cannot easily purchase clay, ordinary earth may be used so long as it is dark, rich soil that has not been farmed-out.

The clay pack *is* prepared much as the water pack, though less cloth should be used so as to permit close contact. When clay *is* to be used for a short period of time and from a reclining position, I have found it advisable to apply it directly to the affected area without a covering material.

ZONE THERAPY: My first contact with zone therapy, an amazing form of natural relief from pain, came some years ago at the Florida sanitorium. A surgeon from the middle west had come to Yungborn to investigate some of the courses of therapy applied by Benedict Lust at that time. He was interested in much of what he had seen and remained far longer than he had originally planned, successfully treating a painful rheumatic condition in his side. One day at lunch he told us this amazing story. Several weeks earlier, he had performed a minor operation. Ether had been used and the surgery was quickly and easily done. Following the operation, the patient was instantly awake, an unnatural condition when ether is used. Investigating, the anesthetist found that the ether tank had ceased operating just as the surgery began, consequently the patient had received no gas. And yet the operation had been painlessly performed!

The surgeon had told this story to several colleagues who refused to believe him. But Dr. Benedict Lust was ready to accept him at his word, the reason being that for many years, zone therapy had been applied at the sanitorium to conditions of extreme pain. Dr. Lust explained that, while the ether had ceased to flow, the pressure which the assistant had applied to the patient's face through the ether mask had been enough to combat the pain of the operation! This was a direct application of zone therapy.

Zone Therapy was first charted by Dr. William Fitzgerald of Hartford, Connecticut arid later outlined by Dr. Benedict Lust in his now famous book on the subject. Credit should also be given to Dr. A. T. Still as being among the first to scientifically note the effects of applied pressure.

Several kinds of instruments are used in the application of zonal pressure. A flat metal object (a broad spoon handle will do) is often used for applying pressure to the nose and mouth in zone one. A small metal comb is sometimes applied to the toes and fingers to eliminate distress in any of the five zones of the body. Where it *is* valuable to apply pressure to the hand or fingers for ten to fifteen minutes, metal clips, shaped much like spring clothes pins, are used. When properly applied, zone therapy has been instrumental in combating the pain of headaches, rheumatics, nerves, hay fever, nausea, earaches and female disorders.

Note that I said zone therapy offers a "natural relief from pain." It does just that without the bad side effects of aspirins, narcotics, etc. but *it is not a cure.* Nature is the only cure.

AFFUSIONS (WATER JETS): Father Kneipp, famed trail blazer in the field of drugless medicine, was among the first to scientifically estimate the value of affusions and the proper application of these natural healers. Affusion is just a fancy word for describing a jet of water. While many had realized the natural good of bathing beneath swiftly running water, Father Kneipp studied the action of these jets upon the body and came to realize two important factors: affusions stimulate the circulation of blood through the body; through this stimulation, affusions can be directed to a specific area of the body to disperse masses of congestion.

The Kneipp course of affusions calls for proper application of the jets to those areas requiring attention. An area of pain is not necessarily the area of congestion, but may only reflect a condition in another part of the body. For this reason, it is necessary to understand the ailment being treated and the Kneipp therapy advised for that condition. The affusion, as practiced by natural therapists, is always cold and delivered at the greatest degree of pressure short of causing pain for the patient.

These jet baths require very little equipment. The water faucet of any sink is in itself a kind of affusion apparatus. How many times have you held your head beneath a tap of running water to alleviate the pain of a headache?

This, in Its simplest form, was an application of the Kneipp principle of healing. To direct the jet at any area of the body, a piece of rubber tubing capable of being fitted over your bathtub faucet can be used. A good focusing nozzle which will permit you to adjust the spray to a fine, powerful jet is obtainable at any hardware store. Believe it or not, these are essentially the pieces of equipment used through the years at Yungborn Sanitoria, where thousands found new health and the joy of life.

FASTING AND ELIMINATION DIETS: The earliest reference to fasting can be found in the Old Testament. Obviously men have fasted from the beginning of time. In a vast number of illnesses, Nature has provided for the fast by simply removing all appetite from the ailing. But fasting cannot be haphazardly applied to all conditions, and even where applied, it must be done with knowledge as well as determination.

The fast and the eliminatory diet serve similar purposes. Each is constructed to clean out the system and return the body to natural balance. I have never gone upon a fast, except where specifically indicated by the nature of the ailment, always preferring the eliminatory diet. "While it is true that the fast will bring about a more rapid cleansing, it is also true that fasting frequently saps the body of energy and must be properly prepared for before-hand.

Even the fast is not a foodless diet. The stomach cries out to be filled and if we do not answer that plea, we will receive little good from fasting. But the true fast can only contain liquid nourishment. Citrus juices, the juices of stewed fruit (prunes, apricots and figs in particular) and herbal teas (non-caffeine) would be a part of your fast. A good practice is to drink a glassful (8 to 10 ounces) of juice each hour of the day. This will help to ease the hunger pains that accompany fasting and will also stimulate elimination.

A hot brew before bedtime and on rising is advisable in the fast, as well as the eliminatory diet. Hot lemonade (prepared with honey or raw sugar) is a pleasant drink. I myself prefer the broth of celery, onions, carrots and spinach, with a bit of vegetable shortening for additional flavor. And, before we forget, cabbage juice is a good broom for sweeping out your insides when fasting or during the eliminatory diet.

There are many eliminatory diets applied around the world and all have had wondrous benefits sworn to them. I have knowledge of some sixteen of these and can substantiate four through personal use. Of these, only two, the grape diet and that which was long practiced at our Yungborn sanitoria in Florida and New Jersey, have proven themselves time and again. I prefer the Yungborn system, but others may choose the grape diet for simplicity and lightning-like speed. The weaknesses of the grape diet lie only in its lack of variety and sudden impact. Some years ago, I traveled about the country on a lecture tour, and found myself eating in every conceivable kind of establishment where vegetables were generally cooked to nothingness and chunks of pork fat were added to the already useless greens and soups. By the end of the tour, I was exhausted beyond the actual strain of the trip. I had momentary spells of dizziness and extreme nausea.

Back home, I put myself upon a grape diet. Within six hours after my return, I consumed three pounds of grapes and a quart of fresh grape juice. And then, as if by magic, the poisonous wastes I had stored up on my trip just poured from me. By nightfall, I was totally recovered and I was able to sleep the night through without the slightest discomfort or restlessness. In short, the grape diet is unpleasant but extremely effective.

The Yungborn diet, on the other hand, is equally effective, though not as fast or dramatic in its impact. The Yungborn diet is pleasant and in no way difficult to adhere to. I have outlined three standard menus for the Yungborn Eliminatory Diet in Chapter 10, as well as simple rules for creating further menus. Study these carefully, for the eliminatory diet is the proverbial friend in need.

It is important for you to realize that each of the following case histories outlined represents an individual who sought natural therapy as a final measure, after a life of unnatural existence, generally including the unbalanced diet, poisoned air, tobacco and alcohol of so-called modern man. The backwardness of such an existence is obvious. The fact that natural therapy was able to help, in even the smallest measure, such cases of decay and debilitation is a true testimonial to the powers of Nature's agents. The fact remains that much of the misery and discomfort suffered by these people would have been avoided through the simple but paramount process of living in harmony with Nature.

In every one of the cases outlined, the first measures taken at the sanitoria involved the three basic steps of natural therapy; Cleanse, Repair, Maintain. The specific treatments used to combat such infection were emergency measures and are rarely needed where a rational life has created natural health. It will serve you better to learn the steps to creating and maintaining natural health, than to invest too much time in studying the symptoms and therapy of each case history out of fear that you may one day need to apply them to your own body. Avoid unnatural excesses! Make of yourself a link in Nature's chain and you will never require cures and convalescence.

ALLERGIES

There is a common practice today, among many physicians, to stamp anything which they cannot successfully diagnose, "allergy." The reason for this is that so little is known about allergies that the diagnosis leaves plenty of room for discussion and explanation. The "indefinite" diagnoses have always been favored by the less responsible physicians. Two hundred years ago, a condition that could not be diagnosed was called "bad humours," and anyone who suffered anything from stomach ache to cancer or gallstones was told his humours were acting up. This was followed by the "acids" theory, where strange and mysterious acids were accountable for all undiagnosed conditions.

This is not to say that allergies do not exist. There certainly is a strange group of body reactions to which has been given the title, allergy. To be exact, there are two such groups; those which are localized on the surface of the body, from face to feet, or skin allergies; and those which inhabit the chest, throat and nasal areas, or respiratory allergies. These two groups include the majority of allergic reactions.

In the respiratory group would be such common conditions as hay fever, asthma, sinusitis, etc. These conditions are centered in the respiratory system, but some (particularly hay fever and sinus conditions) tend to spill over into other areas, as for instance the eyes, which may tear, redden and puff under severe attack. There is good reason to believe that these particular allergies are related to Vitamin C deficiency. Low potency (natural) Vitamin C pills have proven useful in the treatment of such allergies, as has the B complex.

The skin allergies, hives and nettle rash, as an example, are in some degree related to an over-acid condition of the body.

This is not to be confused with the "mysterious acids" of one hundred years ago, which were conveniently blamed for most diseases. The acids I speak of are produced right within the body and consumed day by day in the daily diet. The rational diet, with its balanced intake and natural form, will not support a hyper-acid condition. To defeat this condition when it already exists in the body, it is necessary to cleanse the system completely.

Herbal laxative pills (1-2 a day for three days), mild enemas (1 a day, for a week) and Return to Nature Diet will supply the thorough broom that a hyper-acid condition demands. This is the basis of the Yungborn treatment for skin allergies. The localized treatment prescribed at the sanitorium involved daily natural baths with particular emphasis upon the area affected. Pressure (douche) baths upon the affected area and a mild (not too brisk) rub following the bath, were effective- Where the skin was particularly dry, a few drops of olive oil were applied.

The water used for bathing at Yungborn was excellent but this was not always the case in the areas from which the many patients at the sanitorium came. For that reason, skin allergy patients were instructed to soften the water used for bathing with a cup of starch (such as Linit or any similar product that does not require boiling to dissolve completely in water). Bicarbonate of soda should never be used to soften water for a sensitive skin, since it is an alkali and will have a drying and destructive effect in time.

Dry skin should not be bathed too frequently or for long periods of time. Baths should be quick affairs and olive oil may help to relieve the loss of skin oil. Air baths should be indulged in frequently to substitute for the daily water baths which you may miss.

ANEMIA

Anemia, a condition which has sometimes been described as "blood poverty," is more common, in its various forms, than most would suspect. During an anemic period, the red corpuscles within the system are not being produced quickly enough to replace the normal loss. Since the blood stream is an oxygen-conveyor-belt, carrying the life-giving gas to every part of the body, an insufficient supply of hemoglobin (also symptomatic of anemia) makes it impossible for the body to receive sufficient oxygen. It is for this reason that anemia has often been referred to as slow suffocation.

The absence of sufficient oxygen within the system produces definite outward signs. The anemic patient generally suffers from frequent and severe spells of dizziness, fatigue, listlessness and an inability to concentrate. The anemic patient is frequently forgetful, pale complexioned and easily winded by even moderate physical activity. A combination of these symptoms would more accurately indicate anemia than the famed eye-tissue test (in which the skin immediately beneath the eye is lowered and an examination of the inner tissue, that which lines the eye socket, is performed. In this test, color is used as the determining factor, a red tone supposedly indicating health and a pale tone indicating anemia.)

In addition to the natural regimen (air, sun, water and earth contact) the Yungborn course for anemia specified a diet rich in iron. Particularly vital to this diet and consumed at least once each day were soybeans, liver and unsulphured molasses. Raisins, dried beans, oysters and fresh heart (beef) were included in the daily menu as frequently as possible. These, of course, were consumed in addition to a rational diet of fresh fruits and vegetables and whole grain cereal products. Proper diet and natural living have been sufficient treatment to overcome every case of anemia ever registered at Yungborn. Proof again that it is not Nature who makes healing complex, but man himself.

ARTHRITIS

This condition rarely exists where infection has been prevented from entering the body. Those who suffer from arthritis invariably carry a point of infection within their bodies other than the joint area affected. By combating infection wherever it may arise, in teeth (gums), tonsils, bladder, kidneys, sinuses, appendix or others, you are protecting yourself against a future attack of arthritis.

Vitamin C is an important anti-infection substance. Make certain that your diet contains citrus fruit, green or red pepper, berries and other foods high in the C Vitamin. A diet fortified with the Fountain of Youth Cocktail (See page 152) will never be short of Vitamin C. Mild infections can be overcome with nothing more than an increase in Vitamin C consumption where the diet has undersupplied this important substance. By fortifying your diet with substantial amounts of the C Vitamin and maintaining a natural existence (sun, air, earth and water) you can prevent infection rather than have the more difficult task of curing it once the infection has begun.

T. H. suffered from acute arthritis that brought him to the sanitorium in a semi-crippled state. His left hand was completely immobile and a similar condition had begun at the hips, causing him to bend at the waist when walking, which could only be accomplished with the use of a cane. The pain made sleep almost impossible and for a year he had been using barbituates to induce rest at night.

A three-quarter pack was prescribed to be worn for two hours, twice each week. Cold water rubs were administered each morning with a friction rub of the entire body (the affected area to be rubbed gently to avoid unnecessary pain). Affusions of the knees and the affected area were ordered. The water pressure upon the affected joint was determined by the condition of the patient, the rule being to avoid excess pain at all times.

A non-stimulating diet was ordered, accompanied by the Fountain of Youth Cocktail. Warm compresses were applied at night (heating pads wrapped in wet towels). Sun and air baths were administered daily, weather permitting.

Three weeks after his entrance, T. H. left the sanitorium without the aid of a cane. The pain had not completely abated, but at no time were sleeping pills permitted and after the first night, the patient had slept satisfactorily for the duration of his stay. At home he remained on the non-stimulating diet (fortified with the Fountain of Youth Cocktail) for two months. During that time, he continued the use of warm compresses each night and cold rubs and friction rubs each morning. At the end of two months, the pain had subsided. T. H. then increased the scope of his diet, continuing the emphasis upon Vitamin C foods. One year after he had begun his new life, observing all the laws of natural existence and providing himself with large amounts of Vitamin C foods, the Fountain of Youth Cocktail and brisk wet and friction rubs, T. H. lost all the painful symptoms of arthritis.

BACKACHES

These are among the most inconclusive symptoms of bodily disorders. Backaches may arise from nervous tension, rheumatism, kidney disorders, constipation, colds, foot trouble, insomnia and many more conditions. Here it is important to understand the nature of the pain and any accompanying symptoms. At Yungborn, those complaining of backaches were placed upon non-stimulating diets and daily sun baths with frequent hot compresses upon the affected area until a complete diagnosis could be made.

Where the patient complained of pains in the lower area of the back, on both sides of the spinal column, the kidney, colon or nervous system was invariably found to be the point of danger. In the case of kidney or colon disorders, a day of fasting was prescribed, accompanied by enemas (one quart, 80°, twice daily) and an increased intake of liquids (fruit juices, vegetable broth and water, total of three quarts daily). The hot compresses and sunbaths were continued and a shirt-pack (a shirt of absorbent material, dipped in warm, 85° water) applied before retiring.

Where the patient indicated symptoms of a nervous disposition, the backache was generally found to be induced by the central disorder of the nerves,, Here the treatment of mind and body together was considered primary, in keeping with the adage "a healthy mind in a healthy body." The accompanying symptoms were frequently deceiving, since the patient suffering from acute nervousness may display signs of various conditions which are but surface symptoms. He or she may have false palpitations, though the heart proves to be in excellent condition. The patient may complain of dizziness and unnatural periods of perspiration and overheating, though his or her blood pressure be normal, no trace of anemia, eye or brain disorder present, no apparent cause for fevers, etc.

Where acute nervousness and tension is responsible for the pains, the backache can be temporarily alleviated but final relief lies in the return to and maintenance of a healthy mind and body. Here the backache is symptomatic and treating the symptom is never a successful attack upon the cause of the disorder. However, where the symptom is painful and conducive to further mental strain, it actually contributed to the cause. This is often the case among nervous people. In effect, they induce bodily disorders through the strain upon mind and soul, and the bodily disorders then became a cause for worry that increases the original nervous tension. Here is another cycle, but not one of Nature's doing.

Frequent cold water baths (60°), back affusions, cold neck compresses and air baths were prescribed for the nervous back-ache. Massage proved particularly useful in these cases, with the area of concentration being the lower spinal area, smilingly referred to as the tail-bone. In many such cases, the mere touch of the fingers to this area, where nerve lines come together in a kind of message-center, produced remarkable relief. Kneading the entire spinal column, the trunk of these nerve lines, and stimulating the system through open-handed or slapping strokes, was found soothing. Fountain of 'Youth Cocktail was also prescribed. (See page 152 for formula.)

In all painful conditions resulting from chronic nervous tension, massage has proven effective. The combination of sun-baths, hot compresses, diathermy (electronic heat treatments) and massage are particularly beneficial. However, there is a tendency on the part of many to separate massage or chiropractry (massage therapy) from the whole area of natural healing and to expand upon the importance of this one element. There is no one cure-all in Nature. Any attempt to replace all of Nature's agents with excessive stress upon one area of natural therapy, be it massage, diet, sun bathing or any other, *is* a rejection of the total power of Nature.

The rheumatically induced backache is generally diagnosed through similar rheumatic pains in other areas of the body. It can be assumed that backaches which come and go with extreme temperature and humidity changes, exposure to cold, damp weather without benefit of stimulating and warming exercise, are rheumatic in origin. (See page 122, "RHEUMATICS").

Backaches resulting from localized colds or constipation were treated at Yungborn for those specific causes. Colds that have localized in this area were treated with the general cold therapy applied at the sanitorium, special stress being placed upon sun bathing, hot compresses and the full pack, which was administered nightly until the patient was sufficiently relieved. Massage proved effective in the case of constipation-induced backaches and daily exercises to induce elimination also helped to remove the painful pressure in the lower spinal area.

Most people find it difficult to understand how backaches may arise from foot trouble. It must be explained that the spinal column receives daily punishment from the jouncing flat-footed walk of those who suffer from various foot disorders. The torture boxes within which modern men and women imprison their feet can be held responsible not only for most of the foot trouble of our times, but also for many of the backaches, A daily barefoot tour in garden, yard or field, or even upon the cold tiles of your bathroom, is the first step in reclaiming your foot health. Hot foot baths and massage of the feet and calves, plus a return to natural living have proven their worth countless times in repairing those ravages wrought by man upon himself. Above all, discard your shoes whenever possible. There is no need at all for wearing shoes at home and the sensible person will forget the silly conventions that force these destructive devices upon him sixteen hours a day.

BLADDER INFECTION

L. R. was admitted to Yungborn complaining of the following symptoms: decreased urination, both in the number of urinations each day and the quantity of urine; extreme pain during urination; leg swellings, enlarged pores, particularly of the facial tissue, and a pallid complexion. The condition was diagnosed as an infection of the bladder and a resultant presence of liquid waste matter throughout the system. An eliminatory diet was provided, along with daily full packs to increase elimination through the pores. Clay packs were applied to the lower abdomen for a period of two hours each day, one half hour of which was spent in sun bathing and the remainder in outdoor (shaded) air baths.

Leg packs, to increase elimination, were applied at night and barefoot walks were prescribed daily. All means of increasing elimination, including the use of small enemas, were introduced. The first signs of recovery came three days after the course had begun. L. R. noticed, on removing the leg packs upon the third morning, a marked decrease in the swellings. By the fifth day, the swellings were no longer noticeable, though the leg packs were continued until the tenth day. The return to normal urinary elimination was a day by day process which became noticeable in the second week with increased elimination and lessening of pain during urintion. At the end of two weeks, the patient was discharged. Nature had claimed another victory.

BOILS

The most effective treatment for boils, as practiced at Yungborn, is the clay pack. I have seen these swellings, often the size of a, half-dollar, reduced with amazing speed through the natural therapy of rich earth. The procedure used at the sanitorium was a simple one. A mass of clay about three times the size of the boil, was wrapped in white linen or cotton cloth and applied to the swelling. In one instance, no more than forty-eight hours passed before the boil began to exude a mixture of blood and pus. At this point the cloth was removed and the clay applied directly to the open wound. As the affected area became reduced and cleared of infectious matter, the clay was alternated with cold compresses. Where the boil was not particularly large or painful, cold compresses alone were sufficient to ripen the swelling and clear the toxins.

It is common practice to apply hot compresses to boils. I have known of several such cases and judge, from their outcome, that this is an unwise procedure. The use of heat tends to ripen the swelling unnaturally and, while it quickly opens the infected area, it is not possible to cleanse the area of all the accumulated pus. As a result, in three such cases, boils reappeared shortly either in another area of the body or immediately adjoining the first infection. The eliminatory diet and mild enemas were prescribed for all infections at Yungborn, toward the end of eliminating the store of waste matter that contributes to infection. "When this is combined with the gentle action of earth compresses, the boil is stimulated but not forced into unnatural maturity that leaves pussy matter behind to reform in another area of the body.

In all cases of infection, the standard treatment at Yungborn involved cleansing internally through the use of the enema, externally with natural, air and sun bathing and a completely non-stimulating diet. Fasting accompanied by the Fountain of Youth Cocktail (see page 152) proved effective in severe infection.

CATARACT

The natural treatment of all body disorders lies in the return to Nature through daily living habits and specific attention to the area of injury or infection. The degree of success in natural therapy is dependent on your loyalty to your new life, strict observance of the specific treatment involved, and the degree of degeneration imposed upon your body through unnatural living habits. If you permit decay to go unimpeded, the course of therapy will be a long and difficult one. This is particularly true in disorders involving corrosion, such as ulcers and tuberculosis, and those ending in unnatural growth of tissue, as in cancer and cataract.

In the late stages of cataract, when vision has become severely impaired by the thin coat of tissue that forms across the eye, only the surgeon can bring relief. But surgery itself is not a cure. Once the cataract has been removed by surgery, there is no guaranty that it will not return. Here natural therapy has been successfully employed time and again in retaining eye health. And, in the case of incipient (early) cataract — Nature's agents have halted the growth and finally removed it entirely.

Many programs for counteracting the growth of cataracts have been tried and tested by drugless physicians. That which we found most successful at Yungborn involved syringing the eye itself and affusions of the forehead immediately above the affected eye. A small syringe containing warm (82°) water was used to treat the eye itself, while a strong jet of cold (60°) water trained upon the forehead for a period of three to five minutes, repeated every three hours throughout the day. Cool (68°) foot baths were prescribed and the exclusion of all stimulants, particularly tobacco, liquor and coffee, plus a generally non-stimulating diet was enforced. The results of such treatment proved satisfactory beyond all treatments heretofore employed.

CONSTIPATION

This is possibly the most common ailment of modern man. More important than that, the toxic wastes that accumulate in a constipated system are responsible for a countless number of conditions which are not generally related to digestion or elimination. For this reason, the eliminatory diet (and in acute cases, the fast) is provided as the first measure in most natural therapy no matter where the specific ailment, swelling or infection may appear to be located.

The human body is much like an engine, requiring constant fueling and clearance of the fuel ash. Food is the fuel of the human machine. "When the proper fuel is fed into the furnace (stomach), the machine (heart, blood, lungs and organs) operates efficiently. When poor fuel is fed into the furnace, it will not supply the machinery with needed energy. The fuel is not consumed and remains half-burned within the furnace grate (colon). This half-burned fuel cannot be naturally eliminated and the painful result is called constipation. The related results, the sapping of bodily energy, may result in the infection of any area of the body through the toxic matter that this waste throws into the blood stream.

Laxatives, oils, so-called liver pills, all of these are worthless in treating constipation. Constipation is not a disease of the colon or bowels, but rather of the digestive system. The root of constipation can be found in your refrigerator and on your stove, not in your body. Laxatives attempt to stimulate the peristaltic action (muscles which perform elimination) and induce bowel movements. Instead, they cause the peristalsis to become dependent upon such stimuli and what you then have is a crutch, not a cure. Furthermore, laxatives which are based upon high roughage content, without providing other mineral and vitamin value, will eventually cause grave damage to the stomach and bowels. Many ulcers and ruined digestive systems can be directly traced to heavy consumption of bran. Bran is but one part of the entire wheat stalk. In its natural form, whole grains of wheat will stimulate the eliminatory system without irritating it. The remainder of the wheat product helps to protect us against the bran which, taken alone, will eventually destroy your digestive and eliminatory system. Avoid bran preparations and similar concentrations of roughage.

From a formula many years ago Benedict Lust prepared a compound of some fifteen herbs in the proper balance for stimulating and, at the same time, protecting the eliminatory system against irritation. These herb pills have proven successful in the initial treatment of every case of constipation on record at the Florida and New Jersey sanitoria. If your Health Food Shop does not carry herb pills, you might try concocting your own natural laxative. St. John's Bread, for instance, is such a laxative and is effective in all but the most acute cases.

The following simple recipe will be found to stimulate most common conditions of sluggishness.

NATURE'S OWN FRUIT STIMULANT

   1 lb. dried prunes
   1 lb. dry figs
   1/4 lb. dried unsulphured apricots
   2 quarts of water
   3 lemons, 2 tablespoons of honey

The fruit should not be cooked. It is never necessary to cook dried fruit and such cooking will destroy much of the food value. Simply soak the prunes, figs and apricots in a solution of water and honey into which the lemons have been squeezed and sliced. Allow the fruit to steep overnight. The syrup produced by these fruits is delicious and should be drunk frequently through the day. A heaping plate of Nature's Own Fruit Stimulant each morning will serve to quicken the laggardly pace of your eliminatory system.

The increase in chronic constipation has made its symptoms of nausea, dizziness, fatigue, gaseousness, headaches, and cramps widely known. The growing number of white collar workers and professionals seem to be the central target of constipation. It is obvious that sedentary occupations contribute to systemic sluggishness.

Therefore, increased physical activity is primary in combatting chronic constipation. Walking, swimming and bowling are three perfect sports in overcoming sluggishness. Calisthenics, with particular emphasis on knee bends and other toe touching exercises, are equally effective. Healing should never be an uncomfortable or annoying process. The most successful form of physical activity is that which not only attacks the point of infection, but also brings pleasure and satisfaction. Here again the value of tending mind and body at one and the same time is obvious and appreciable.

Both acute and chronic constipation can only be ended through wise food habits and constant: attention to bowel movements. The constipation sufferer cannot hope to attain regularity without providing a program of regularity for his eliminatory system. Once the cleansing and maintenance of a healthy digestive system has begun, you must provide a definite hour of the day for evacuation and you must keep that appointment as regularly as you keep your office hours or your radio listening habits. Morning hours, following the two large meals of the preceding day, are best. But morning, noon and night, consistency is demanded. You must not fool your system, for in the end it is yourself who is being tricked.

The idea that all men and women must maintain the same eliminatory habits is a mistaken approach to natural therapy. Nature goes to great lengths to preserve individuality. In a pail of snow, containing billions of snowflakes, no two snowflakes appear alike under the microscope. No two eliminatory systems are exactly alike. Where one person may require two and possibly three bowel movements a day, another will find need for no more than one each day. Individuality, not comformity, is the law of nature.

Neither acute nor chronic constipation can be completely alleviated without first cleansing the system. Though the source of sluggishness is in your diet, the waste matter accumulated through improper nutrition cannot be eliminated merely by adopting sane eating habits. If a pipeline, meant to carry water, is suddenly flooded with oil, you will not clean that pipe merely by sending water through it once more. The pipe must be scoured out with an oil-solvent at the same time as the intake of oil is halted and replaced with water. In the same way, chronic constipation can only be ended by three simultaneous procedures.

1.   Cleansing the intestines through internal baths (enemas).
2.   Restoring the digestive system to health through first an eliminatory diet and then a balanced food program.
3.   Incorporating Nature's agents, air and natural baths particularly, in your daily life.

K. R. was a woman of fifty-two who had suffered from chronic constipation for eight years. "When she registered at Yungborn, in New Jersey, she complained of headaches, dizziness, loss of appetite, intermittent cramps and general fatigue. She was underweight (though this is not common to chronic constipation) and sallow skinned, with deep lines of fatigue etched upon her face. The discomfort she had known all those years made sleeping difficult and threatened to create an acute condition of insomnia.

In addition to the eliminatory diet and daily air baths, warm (80°) natural baths were prescribed, accompanied by abdominal massages. Increased physical activity, sleeping-out and a one-a-day enema administered at nine in the morning, were also ineluded in her treatment. The enema was warm (72°) and no more than ten ounces (a large water glass). Since K. R.'s condition was chronic and of a long history, it was necessary to administer a larger enema than is usually demanded and to begin each bowel movement with these internal baths. In less serious cases a smaller bath (about 4 to 6 ounces, or half a water glass) was generally prescribed to *follow* bowel movements and serve to increase the effectiveness of the movement. K. R.'s condition, however, demanded that each movement be induced through an enema which she retained for ten to fifteen minutes simply by lying upon her stomach for that period of time. These small enemas are called retentive enemas. However, a major internal bath (1 pint) was given the first day. This major enema is not retained and the lying down process is unnecessary here.

In three days, it was no longer necessary to induce bowel movements and the internal bath was only used following the evacuation to help cleanse any remaining waste from the intestines. However, noticeable improvement occurred in less than that time. By the second day, K. R.'s appetite increased under the ministrations of the beautiful surroundings of the New Jersey hills, daily air and natural baths and a wholesome eliminatory diet which was expanded each day to accommodate her thriving appetite. Her natural baths were taken in the evening and abdominal pack was donned following the bath and prior to retiring. A pitcher of water was placed at her bed to help her increase liquid intake. Beyond these, the only remaining therapy was the deep knee bend exercise to be performed prior to the internal bath each morning.

K. R. left the sanitorium two weeks after she had entered. It may interest you to know that among the prescriptions for future treatment given her upon leaving was the cryptic note, "Fire your domestic worker." K. R.'s condition grew largely from her sedentary life. The daily exertion of light house work, stooping, dusting, sweeping, etc., was not a part of her life. It is to be doubted that K. R.'s domestic worker suffered from constipation. And I can tell you that having returned to a life of rational eating, employment of Nature's agents and daily exercise, K. R. is no longer a member of the chronic constipation club. In nine years now she has had but half a dozen brief spells of acute sluggishness, most of those within the first year. A small enema and one week of eliminatory dieting was all that was needed to end those.

COUGHS

The cough is deceptive but an important sign of sickness. It was obviously designed to warn you against impending danger, for the cough itself is not a disease, but the outward signal of disease. Coughs are in fact reactions to nerve signals set up in the body and the transmitter of that signal may lie in the stomach, chest, lungs, etc. Possibly the three most common causes of the cough are bronchial and lung irritation (a common complaint of the smoker and of those living in and about industrial areas where chemical smokes are constantly inhaled), chest colds and tuberculosis.

B. J., a patient at the Florida sanitorium, suffered from a constant, hacking cough. He was a heavy smoker and chest colds had become a chronic ailment of his. At first he was troubled with winter colds which disappeared in April or the beginning of May. Later, he began catching summer colds and colds that lasted until September or October. After a while, he ceased calling them by name, for the colds became year 'round affairs.

In this case, as will frequently occur, the patient was well aware of the major cause of his distress. He was as fond of his cigar as he was of his wife, possibly fonder. B. J. smoked some fourteen to sixteen cigars a day. Though we will talk at length about the dangers of tobacco in a later chapter, I would like to state two simple statistics at this point. Dr. Frederick B. Flinn of New York found that in 100 smokers, who averaged twenty-eight cigarettes a day, 73 suffered throat congestion, 66 coughs, 7 irritation of the throat. Dr. Emil Bogen, in a similar test, found thirty with mouth irritations and thirty with coughs. This is just a small indication of the toxicity of tobacco.

B. J. knew that much of his pain (persistent coughs can be extremely painful) was a direct result of tobacco, but still he persisted in smoking. Though the rules at Yungborn permitted a good deal of personal choice, they specifically forbid smoking, moderate or otherwise. We are opposed to slow suicide as we are to jumping from tall buildings. Therefore, B. J. was refused admittance to the sanitorium twice. The third time, after his pledge to throw away the smoking habit, he was admitted for treatment.

The course of therapy outlined was simple at first. A series of enemas, natural baths, air baths and an eliminatory diet, lasted for three days. At the end of that time, the cough was completely eliminated. In addition to the eliminatory diet of raw fruits and non-leguminous (no beans or potatoes) vegetables, an increased amount of fluids was ordered for B. J., with a glass of fruit juice or plain water to be taken each hour. Moistening of the dry throat tissues after each cough with a swallow or two of water or fruit juices was prescribed. A hot fruit drink, both morning and night, was also ordered.

TWENTY-FOUR HOUR COLD COURSE

The cold, which was in part responsible for the cough, had to be eliminated before the cough itself could be relieved. Here the Twenty-four Hour Cold Course was used. B. J. was wrapped in a luke-warm wet terry cloth bathrobe, the kind often used for beach wear. Around the wet pack, a heavy woolen blanket was placed and B. J. bedded down for the night. The outer layer was changed twice during the evening to keep the patient completely warm, and constant intake of liquids (two quarts of fruit and vegetable juices or water) completed the course. At two in the morning (six hours after the pack has been placed upon him) the patient awoke and asked to be allowed to leave the

bed. The cold had broken. The pack was removed and dry bedding was substituted. The Twenty-Four Hour Cold Course had done its job, and in a quarter of the maximum time provided for.

During the remainder of his stay, B. J. was provided with a diet largely consisting of citrus fruits and green vegetables and no starchy foods were permitted. All beverages were heated and he showed a particular fondness for vegetable broth. The mild residue of catarh that remained in nose and throat were quickly cleansed with a salt water solution that he sniffed and gargled four times each day. Most important were the air baths, which hardened his system against recurrent colds. Foot baths were prescribed (about 70°) and daily exercise upon stone or tile to stimulate circulation in the feet. These, and only these, were all that were needed to deliver B. J. from a painful and enervating condition that had plagued him for over ten years.

DIABETES

L. R. J. came to the sanitorium one summer morning complaining of a violent increase in appetite, an unquenchable thirst and increased fatigue. It was also noted that the patient was constipated, showed an unusual hardness of skin tissues and complained of a constant dryness of the throat and mouth and persistent indigestion. An analysis of L. R. J.'s urine was immediately ordered. As had been expected, the analysis proved the presence of a high degree of sugar. Diabetes!

L. R. J. was immediately ordered into a steam bath. These baths were repeated three times a week. At the end of each bath, the patient was dried with a thick, coarse towel rubbed briskly across the body until the friction of towel upon skin produced a pleasant warmth. Luke-warm (73 degrees) abdominal compresses were applied each night and the friction rub was repeated upon arising.

A non-stimulating, unseasoned (salt and sugarless) diet was ordered and sternly administered. Mild enemas were provided once each day. Special stress was placed upon air contact, with outdoor exercise (mild) and daily walks prescribed. L. R. J. left the sanitorium six weeks after he had entered, the persistent thirst and hunger removed and with a rediscovery of his natural energy. Diabetes had been conquered by Nature.

DIZZINESS

Here again is a sympton of decay which is often mistaken for the condition itself. Dizziness may be an outward sign of such varied conditions as anemia (blood poverty), liver disorders, high blood pressure, low blood pressure, colds, menstruation, rheumatics and more. The point to be made here is that there is no cure for dizziness,, for a sympton cannot be cured. The heaving, whirling, nauseating sensation of dizziness can be alleviated. But a permanent cure can only be had when the underlying cause has been discovered and attended to.

M. R. suffered from repeated spells of dizziness. The first attack had come two years before he had registered at Yungborn. He had been sitting in a deep, upholstered chair late one afternoon when his wife called from another room. He rose quickly from the chair and was suddenly seized with a dull throbbing sensation at the temples that gave way to a spinning, enveloping blackness. He attempted to take a single step forward and sank to the floor.

Following that initial attack, M. R. was repeatedly the victim of dizziness, nausea, physical unbalance and collapse. A full examination was made of the patient upon his entrance into Yungborn, and he was found to be suffering from exceedingly high blood pressure. A long range course was outlined to deal with this and, I might add, proved successful. But the immediate symptoms, nausea, dizziness, etc., were dealt with at once.

Luke-warm foot baths were applied daily, followed by cold knee and thigh affusions. Stimulating foot and leg packs were applied before sleep and a water rub-down (70 degrees) upon rising. A non-stimulating diet (see page 180) was ordered as well as prolonged barefoot walks and air baths. Neck massage and repeated cold packs were advised during the first day of treatment in the event of attack. These were discarded shortly, since they were no longer needed. The attacks had subsided and, with the return of a healthy constitution, were gone completely.

Again I must repeat, each case of dizziness must be treated as a symptom of more serious causes and the alleviation of dizziness itself is not a cure of such underlying illness. Find out what the root of your dizziness is and attack the root, not the leaf.

EAR ACHES

M. S. came to the sanitorium with symptoms that gravely disturbed him. For over a year, his left ear had been strangely affected; buzzing and ringing sounds occurred, pain sometimes accompanying them, and his left ear was rapidly losing its hearing. He painfully feared the worst — deafness! Sounds serious, does it not? And indeed it was, for M. S. It continued to be serious for a full three minutes after he arrived, following which a small, hooked, stainless-steel tool was placed in his left ear (no anesthesia required) and a plug of ear wax, about one-third of an inch long, was removed. The ear was irrigated with a stream of warm water from a ball syringe. That was the end of the buzzing and ringing and the end of M. S.'s fears. Full hearing was instantly restored.

Ear wax has a natural function and its presence is not a cause for alarm. Daily washing and frequent syringing of the ears has always protected me against an over-deposit of the ear wax. Above all, let me warn against probings of the ear with pins, toothpicks, letter openers and other haphazard weapons. Such random expeditions can lead to serious injury of the delicate membranes that lie behind the concha (external ear).

When ear noises occur on one side only, wax is almost always the cause. The treatment, as in the case of M. S., is obvious. When the noises occur in both ears the cause is more serious and may frequently be traced to anemia, and high blood pressure. Where these were found to be the root cause, the sanitorium treatment did not revolve around the ears but concentrated on the specific anemia (since there are numerous forms) or the blood pressure. At Yungborn special diets were important factors in treating these two, and I have reproduced examples of such diets in Chapters 9 and 10.

In a great number of patients examined at Yungborn, I noticed that where the complaint was of noises in the ears there was a common fear of mental instability. This is a serious error that arises from the belief that all sounds heard by one person and unheard by others present are an indication of approaching insanity. The ringing or buzzing sounds are here being confused with the "hidden voices" of the unstable. Where such a mis-understanding exists, worry and constant fear of approaching insanity can cause serious shock to the nervous system. Be assured yourself that there is no direct relationship between the buzzing sounds of anemia, high blood pressure, etc., and the accuser voices of insanity. And spread this news where it may do the most good.

Excessive drinking, smoking and the use of such "harmless" drugs as aspirin and quinine are often responsible for ear noise. Here the choice is obvious: give up liquor, tobacco and drugs or content yourself with a life of intermittent ringing and buzzing sounds.

A. T., a young woman who had suffered from excessive earaches for almost a year had given up all hope of relief and came to Yungborn for a general rest. Persistent ear aches had stolen all happiness from her and her personality was devoid of joy or vitality. She moped about the grounds- of the sanitorium, forlorn and hopelessly resigned to a torturous fate.

A non-stimulating diet was prescribed (Chapter 10), ear compresses (72 degrees) were applied, and baths of the ear and surrounding region administered at three-hour intervals. Abdominal packs were worn at night and natural baths were a morning course. Jets of water were introduced into the ear with a small syringe and retained by cocking the head to one side or resting it upon a pillow. The jet brought quick relief and, when pain returned, the ear was emptied by simply raising the head and the process repeated several times.

Within a week the pain had subsided sufficiently to create tremendous, personality changes. A. T. returned to a natural capacity for gay and active living. It was as though she had been reborn.

The mild but lingering ear pains were now treated with zone therapy. In inflammation of the ear, loss of hearing (where the tissues themselves have not become withered or injured), ear aches, etc., the zone under attack is number five. In all cases where zone therapy is to be applied to ear conditions, zone five is the area of treatment by zone therapists, Some practitioners treat ear pains with pressure upon the small finger of the corresponding hand or the small toes of the corresponding foot, both lying within the fifth zone.

Massage of the same areas is preferred by others, an aluminum or steel comb being used for the purpose. The steel comb is a much used instrument among zone therapists.

In the case of A. T., pressure was introduced through the mouth and directly below the affected ear. A tenaculum (small stainless steel bar with a curved head) was placed beneath the last tooth and pressure brought to bear below the area of pain. I clocked the entire procedure. In less than five minutes, pressure was removed and the pain ceased to exist. This procedure was repeated several times when pain returned. Each recurrence was less painful than the last and the period of time between each attack lengthened. It was finally possible for the patient to treat herself through the simple device of biting down upon a small (half-inch) wad of cotton in the same area of the mouth treated previously. In six weeks, A. T. reported to the sanitorium that the pain had been totally relieved.

EYES

Eye irregularities are generally of two categories: infections or muscular incapacities. While a condition such as cataract is a growth and therefore an exception to the rule, it is none the less true that the majority of eye ailments are either of muscular or infectious origin. All infections treated at Yungborn received a general program of therapy plus specific treatment for the area in which the infection had localized. The application of the anti-infection program differed only in degree from one infection to another. The final aim always remained the same, the internal and external cleansing of the body.

C. K., a woman in her middle thirties, had, since childhood, been the victim of repeated eye infections. When she entered the sanitorium both eyes were severely affected, red-rimmed, containing a yellow discharge which encrusted upon the eyelids each night and made it impossible for her to open her eyes each morning without first wetting them and removing the caked discharge. The eyes were extremely sensitive to light and vision was markedly impaired. She was suffering from an advanced form of conjunctivitis (commonly called "pink-eye.")

An eliminatory diet was ordered. During the first three days full (one quart at 80 degrees) enemas were ordered. These were later exchanged for small (a drinking glass full of 72 degrees) enemas taken each morning. A three-quarter (neck to thighs) pack was applied for half an hour each day followed by a hip bath (86 degrees). Hot baths and applications (96 degrees) were applied each morning and throat and calf compresses before retirement. The eyes were bathed with cold (60 degrees) water every three hours each day. At the start of the second week, the eye infection cleared and several small boils appeared upon the back. The toxins had been forced into a new exit. The treatment was continued, with cold (60 degrees) compresses applied to the boils which opened quickly. C. K. was discharged after ten days with instructions to remain upon a non-stimulating diet and continue daily eye baths and short sun baths. That was twelve years ago and the condition has never returned.

Treatment for muscular incapacities differs greatly from that prescribed for infection. While eye baths (60 degrees) are ordered for both, the treatment for muscular weaknesses would of course be aimed at strengthening and rebuilding the deteriorated muscle tissue. The major eye weaknesses that have become common with the general increase in detailed work, sewing, reading, etc., are the result of muscular irregularities. While the tendency toward shortened or stretched eye muscles can be inherited and exaggerated through improper eye care, this tendency can also be combated through a natural program of eye care and strengthening.

The natural method for rebuilding weakened or strained eye muscles revolves around muscular exercise, rest and proper diet. The somewhat recent discovery that Vitamin A is a deterrent to night blindness and other eye disorders has caused some to turn to carrot juice and other foods rich in the A Vitamin as some cure-all for eye defects. Even if diet could be considered a cure-all (and Nature indicates to us that diet is but one important component of a program for natural health), it would still be a serious mistake to isolate one food value and turn to it as an answer to disease and decay. If the eye muscles have become weakened, they must be fed not only with Vitamin A, but with a balanced diet that also stresses the B Complex, that family of foods that protects and strengthens muscular and nerve tissue.

Rest and protection must be guaranteed for the eyes. Protecting the eyes involves such simple but basic steps as reading only under conditions that will not create an exaggerated amount of strain. Reading in itself is not a natural process, but the knowledge of mankind lies within the books of the libraries of the world and must be conserved and continued. This rather recent practice (reading is, at most, five thousand years old, while man has between five hundred thousand and a million years of history behind him) makes it necessary for all of us to take special precautions to protect our eye health. You know the proper method for reading but the question is, how often do you follow it. Do you make certain that there is enough light upon the page of your book before you begin to read? Do you hold the book at least two hand spans (fingers extended) from your eyes? Do you read from a sitting position, the book supported firmly in your hands to avoid constant motion of the reading matter upon which your eyes are focusing? If so, you are protecting your eyes. Reading without proper light; holding the reading matter immediately before your *eyes so* that they are forced to constantly strain the muscles for proper focus; reading in bed with the printed matter swaying and bobbing with each breath you take, thus forcing the eyes to focus and refocus a hundred times a minute, all of these are the stones that pave the road to impaired vision.

Providing the proper reading conditions and working conditions will not return the eyes to health once that health has been injured. Here diet, exercise and hygiene take over. Eye hygiene, as already stated, requires daily cold baths for the eyes. Frequent rest periods for the eyes, particularly during reading or close work, are also primary to their health. Do not wait for your *eyes* to tell you that they are tired. If your eyes signal through pain, tearing or dizziness that they have been strained, then you have waited too long to supply needed rest. Make it a rule to rest your *eyes* at least twice a day under any circumstances. If you are reading or using your eyes for unusually close work, apply a half-hour rule to your program of rest. Never work more than thirty minutes at a time without using the following simple steps for eye rest:

1. PALMING. Close both *eyes* and rest the palms of the hands lightly upon them. Slowly roll the eyes within the sockets in wide circles which take the eye-balls to the extreme walls, roof and floor of the eyes. Repeat this roll a dozen times or more.

2. MASSAGE. Follow the palming with massage. While

the eyes remain closed, place the thumb and forefinger of one hand upon the eyelids and rotate slowly with a gentle pressure that brings comforting relief.

3. CLAMPING. Now clamp the lids of your eyes together as tightly as you are able, and then open them wide. Repeat this lid exercise half a dozen times.

No matter what the condition of your eyes, this program of relaxation is basic to protecting your sight,, Where the eyes have already lost the muscular capacity to afford fine vision, you may be interested in the program of exercise evolved at Yung-born. This program was intended to strengthen the weakened muscles of the eyes and had, as its final aim, the elimination of eye glasses. But it must be explained that full sight could never be attained even with the program applied at the sanitorium so long as the patient continued to depend upon eyeglasses for visual support. If he or she was merely interested in stopping the loss of visual capacity then it was possible to do so without removing the glasses. But where the patient was determined to return to a total state of eye health and full visual capacity it was necessary that the glasses be discarded before the program was begun.

YUNGBORN SIGHT STRENGTHENING PROGRAM:

Diet and all of the components of natural living must be observed. Cleanse the system, feed the body for health, not merely to satisfy taste buds. Sun, air, and natural baths must be a part of your daily life. These basic requirements satisfied, the Yungborn Sight Strengthening Program may be applied. These exercises were prescribed twice daily at the sanitorium, on arising and prior to retiring for the night. The only piece of equipment used for these exercises consisted of a small card (about three inches square) upon which a black circle about the size of a dime had been drawn. Each exercise was applied first to one eye, while the other remained closed, then alternated and finally both eyes completed the exercise.

1. Holding the card a hand span (ten inches) from the eyes, the focus is drawn first to the black circle upon the card and then to an object five or more feet away. This shifting of focus *is* done quickly and repeated twenty times with each eye and twenty times with both. This motion from the near focal point upon the card to another at many times the distance strengthens the eye muscles through swift, vigorous action.

2. Holding the card one inch from the face and concentrat ing upon the black focal point, the card is moved from a point immediately above the eyes to one below the chin while each eye is alternately opened and moved from top to bottom in pur suit of the focal point. Twenty times for each eye and twenty for both *is* the minimal course of exercise.

3. Holding the card one inch from the face, it is moved from one side of the face to the other as the eyes are moved in changing focus with the card; ten times per eye and ten for both.

4. At a distance of six inches, the card is rotated five times clock-wise and five counter-clock-wise for each eye and the same for both.

5. At a distance of one inch, the card is moved from left side of forehead to right side of chin and then from right of chin to left of forehead, forming an X in the air, while the eyes, alternately and then together, move quickly in diagonal lines of pursuit.

These five exercises practiced twice a day, plus a program of rest and natural existence, have brought new strength and life to thousands. Treasure your eyes, for they are the windows of your soul.

FATIGUE

Nowhere is the truth that mind and body are one more clearly-exhibited than in the case of chronic fatigue. Temporary fatigue is easily traced to a lost night's sleep, an unusual amount of physical labor, etc. Chronic fatigue, however, is not merely a matter of bodily wear and exertion. How many people do you know who constantly complain of fatigue though their regular day's labor is not at all excessive? How many times have you found yourself suffering from exhaustion at a time when you were even less physically active than usual? Mind and body demand activity, and attention to one without exercise of the other may lead to exhaustion of both. I have known few people who maintain a well balanced daily program of mental and physical activity who suffered from chronic fatigue.

As in all other cases, fatigue was treated at Yungborn first with a program for natural living. Air, sun, water and earth can never be omitted from a natural program for health. Fatigue occurs more frequently among people who oversleep. Late risers are common victims of chronic tiredness. Indoor workers and livers complain of a constant lack of energy. And starchy diets tend to support this condition. The Yungborn course for fatigue eliminated all of these, stressing early bed habits, both retiring and rising. The lights at Yungborn rarely burned past ten at night and few slept beyond six. Balanced diets, with particular emphasis on nerve and energy foods were prescribed for this condition, with increased consumption of Vitamin B complex, iron, and particularly in hot weather, mineral salts.

Boredom was avoided like the plague. Patients were urged and assisted in busying themselves most of the day with physical and mental activity that kept them in full tone. But such activities were always productive, not senseless motion for the sake of motion. How much better it is to gain your exercise from planting, weeding and harvesting a vegetable garden than from repetitious knee bends and toe touching exercises. Motion-to-ward-creation is an underlying law of Nature.

The natural program to alleviate chronic fatigue also involves daily cold (60 degrees) baths and chest and back affusions. The affusions proved particularly successful and were used to alleviate the aches and pains of unused muscles even while increased activity was provided for those muscles. Compresses brought quick relief when applied nightly to the sore and weary portions of the body. Fountain of Youth Cocktail prescribed daily. (See page 152.)

Most important of all natural methods in alleviating fatigue is the use of air and earth contact. Barefoot walks in shorts or sun suits when weather permits and outdoor activity all year round proved the surest course of satisfying the body needs that induce fatigue.

FEET

A popular cry among the American GI's in World War II was "Oh, my aching back." But a more accurate phrase might have been, "Oh, my aching feet." It is estimated that roughly seventy percent of all our countrymen suffer from some foot disorder, including club feet, fallen arches, ingrown toenails, corns, athletes' foot, blisters, swellings, etc.

Though there are no statistics concerning the foot health of early Americans, it *is* safe to presume that nowhere near the present percentage of foot sufferers existed two hundred years ago, when much of America lived upon the farm and barefoot walking was the rule six days a week. Almost all of the present day foot ills can be directly traced to man's effort to force twenty-six bones and some thirty cubic inches of blood and tissue into the torturous confines of string, steel and leather called a shoe. Corns, calluses and blisters became the rule as men and women cramped healthy feet into these leather prisons. Overlapping toes, athletes foot and ingrown toenails were the direct result of squeezing the feet into confining quarters and denying the air and sun that would protect them.

The two worst public enemies manufactured in the shoe factories are the high heeled shoes and the rubber and canvas affair worn by athletes. It is no accident that "athletes foot" takes its name from those men who spend long hours in sneakers. Footwear that permits no ventilation holds the toxic discharge of the foot tissue and creates the atmosphere necessary for the growth of fungi. In addition to this unhealthy state, the rubber soled shoe or sneaker acts to insulate the wearer from the benefits of earth contact. Thus, while these shoes create the conditions that contribute to decay, they also isolate the feet from one of the natural agents which would ordinarily serve to strengthen the feet against such decay.

The high heeled shoe, as we have already mentioned, is directly responsible for many of the bodily aches and pains that pursue the modern woman. The twisting and bobbing action of a body that is forced to walk upon these wood and leather stilts creates immeasurable damage to muscle, bone and nerve from head to toe. But worst of all is the effect of these monstrous devices upon women's feet. By bending the feet into semi-permanent positions of unnatural distortion, the high heeled shoes succeed in destroying the natural forms and muscular strength of the feet. No false pride or fashion fetish can excuse this deliberate sabotage of bodily health.

It is quite possible, even in our present society, for the average person to spend several hours each day in barefoot walk, work and exercise. It is also a simple matter for all of us, even during the working day, to shoe our feet in unconfining wear that will permit the skin to receive the benefit of air. Sandals, preferably wooden or leather soled, and the perforated and woven Mexican type shoe permit such constant benefits. When at home, in the garden or yard, make certain that your feet receive the strengthening and invigorating stimulus of barefoot exercise and earth contact. Whenever possible, avoid the use of confining footwear.

The natural therapy for bunions, blisters and calluses is the same as that for corns. But it is important to realize that none of these conditions can be permanently alleviated without doing away with the source of irritation. Unless you are willing to carry on an endless campaign against such painful conditions, you had better eliminate the source, the improper footwear you have forced upon your innocent feet.

In addition to perverting the natural form of the foot, most shoes tend to immobilize many of the foot muscles provided by Nature. This condition reduces the perfect mechanism provided us at birth to a condition of degeneration through disuse. Without proper exercise the muscles that support a healthy foot fall into a decline that brings with it foot fatigue, pain and a loss of stability. Realizing this, Yungborn created an effective program for returning aching and weakened feet to a condition of natural health. This consisted of hot baths, cold water rubs, massage and, most important of all, exercise. These were developed not only to strengthen the muscles of the feet but those of the legs and back which support our daily foot work, thus helping to eliminate the leg and back pains that often originate in the feet. It is important to remember in these, as in all exercises, that the patient's capacity for such stimulation was always ascertained before the exact program of exercise was provided. Never guide yourself according to the abilities or constitution of others, but provide for yourself what you can best afford and from which you will most benefit. To each his own.

1.   The first exercise is performed from a face-up reclining position. The arms are outstretched and with the palms of the hands and the toes of the feet the body is raised. From this position, the body is moved slowly forward and backward from a tip-toe position to a point at which the heels almost touch the ground. This is repeated some ten or fifteen times.

2.   Fingers touching the ground and one leg extended well behind the other in the position of a track runner, the balance of the body is moved first from the toes of one foot to the toes of the other. This shifting is repeated another ten to fifteen times. Both of these first two exercises are extremely beneficial to feet and legs, and to back muscles.

3.   Taking a book or a strong box no more than three inches thick, the patient stands upon it so that the front half of the foot extends over the edge. Now, moving slowly forward and then backward, the toes are made to touch the ground and then return.

4.   Now the position is reversed, with the heels extending over the edge and the swaying repeated. This time the heels are made to touch the ground and return. Both of these exercises will help to strengthen the arches and calf muscles.

5.   Holding on to a chair or table for balance, the body is supported upon the toes of one foot. In the fashion of a ballet dancer, the raised leg is moved first forward and then backward to the highest degree obtainable. The true feeling of ballet grace can be attained if the free leg is swung in a slow and wide arc front to back. The legs are to be alternated during the exercise.

6.   Standing upon the toes of both feet, the body is revolved slowly.

7.   Lying flat on the back, the legs are raised one at a time and the toes and ankles stretched as far forward as possible. If the patient is particularly eager and relatively well toned, he or she may attempt to raise both legs simultaneously without bending the knees and then perform the exercise. This is no small feat, but well worth the effort.

8.   Standing upon the outer rim of the feet, the patient walks briskly about. Following this, the position is shifted to the inner rim of the feet and the brisk walk repeated.

These are all the exercises provided in the Yungborn Foot Health program. You will notice that no pencil-lifting or marble rolling or the like is included. Oddly enough, many so-called experts have concocted exercises which a normally healthy foot would find difficult to perform, and then demanded that sore and suffering feet run them through without faltering. What these people fail to realize is that the patient would not turn to them for assistance if he could perform such herculean feats of calisthenics. Exercises that are beyond the immediate ability o^ the patient always tend to discourage him or her and in the end, defeat the original purpose. The success or failure of a program of exercise is decided by the regularity with which the program *is* practiced. Anything that tends to discourage regular practice is undesirable no matter how beneficial its final effects might promise to be.

FIBROID TUMOR

Among the most painful and dangerous of female disorders is the fibroid tumor of the uterus. In part, the danger is psychological rather than physical. The increased incidence of cancer together with a wide publicity campaign, has made the public highly cancer-conscious. For this reason, the discovery of almost any tumor on the body will generally strike terror into the heart of the strongest person. Thus the relatively common fibroid tumor which attacks the uterus is often mistaken for a malignant tumor (cancer), and the resultant shock is almost as destructive as the growth itself.

Since the possibility of cancer always exists where an unnatural growth is discovered, it is important that the patient be immediately examined. Time is essential, since medical science has made great strides in the treatment of cancers which have been detected in an early stage. Learn these signs of possible cancer by heart:

1. Constant bleeding despite efforts to staunch the flow.
2. Repeated and severe attacks of indigestion.
3. Sudden growth or change in shape of a mole, birthmark, etc.
4. Discoloration of stool (bowel movement).
5. Painful or sore lump or spot on or beneath the skin which refuses to heal.

As for the fibroid tumor of the uterus, this may be the size of a pea or smaller and may grow to the size of a lemon or larger. Though it originates in the uterus, the tumor may grow into the uterine cavity during its maturation.

As the tumor develops the uterus becomes knobby and enlarged. Pressure of the growth upon the bladder may bring pain and increased urination. Conversely, fibroid tumors often induce constipation through pressure upon the rectum. Hemorrhaging is a frequent tumor warning. The existence of a fibroid tumor within the uterus is often a cause of natural abortion (miscarriage).

At Yungborn, such growths were treated through natural baths, diet, wet wraps and therapeutic gymnastics. A daily lukewarm *(77* to 82 degrees) bath was prescribed with cold compresses to be applied to the vagina at bedtime. Sexual intercourse and other activities which might aggravate the condition were strictly forbidden. As in most instances, the Yungborn regimen for fibroid tumors also involved the Return to Nature Diet. A half pack (abdomen to feet) was applied for one hour each day and thigh and spinal douches (pressure baths) were prescribed three times weekly.

Exercises (therapeutic gymnastics) were provided for the patient, though sports which provided entertainment and a lift to the morale were always preferred to ordinary exercise. Thus, while the bicycle exercise (in which the patient lies upon her back and lifts the body from the waist, propelling the legs as though bicycling) proved effective in treating tumors of the uterus, actual bicycling was encouraged. In a like manner, if the patient acknowledged a fondness for rowing, this sport was prescribed rather than a similar exercise such as sit-ups (in which the patient lies flat, hands locked behind head, and lifts and lowers the body from waist to head without shifting the feet).

Other exercises recommended were the waist twist (from an upright position, hands behind head, the body is twisted from extreme right to extreme left and back again without moving the feet); deep knee bends, toe touching and the scissors exercise (from prone position raise legs and then move slowly apart and together as though a scissors).

Since fibroid tumors may exist for many years without making themselves known to the patient, and since tumors of the uterus are particularly common among women at menopause (change of life), it would seem a wise precaution if every woman adopted much of this program from age forty on.

GALL BLADDER INFECTIONS

The Yungborn program for alleviating the pain of gall-stones and gall bladder infections involves a complete cleansing of the system. A three day fast involving the intake of no solid foods and a quart of Fountain of Youth Cocktail daily was the standard beginning treatment. For gall bladder conditions the Fountain of Youth Cocktail was reinforced with the liquid derived from an additional four tablespoons of wheat germ and a cup of chopped kale or carrot tops. These increased intake of Vitamins K and E, generally found deficient in gall bladder conditions.

The first day of treatment, the patient was internally cleansed with a full enema and a two hour steam bath. For two days following a small enema was continued once a day. Abdominal compresses were prescribed during the night. Sun baths were an important part of the treatment, as were abdominal exercises; deep knee bends, body twists and the like, to stimulate and tone the abdominal area. The steam bath was continued on the second and third day, this time for periods of one hour a day.

On the fourth day, lean meats, eggs or fish, twice daily, were added to the diet, and steam baths were discontinued. In their place, warm (80 degrees) natural baths were prescribed nightly and cold rubs each morning. The friction rub was observed twice daily, following the morning cold rub and the evening natural bath.

On the tenth day, the non-stimulating diet was prescribed. Abdominal compresses were continued as well as morning cold rubs and evening natural baths, and daily sun baths. Abdominal exercise and massage was a daily requirement throughout the program.

I have seen the above program dramatically prove its true value in more than a dozen cases of serious bladder infection at Yungborn sanitoria. Nature has provided a wonderful course of therapy for all bladder infections, if only men will be wise enough to recognize and use this great gift.

HEADACHES:

The causes of headaches are many and it is always advisable to understand the root of all head pains before attempting to counteract them. Since such pains are Nature's means of warning us of internal disturbances, it is unwise to attempt to treat the headache alone, but rather to understand its origin and treat both cause and symptom.

Among the most common conditions creating headaches can be listed eye strain, stomach disorders, menstruation, hunger, high blood pressure, rheumatics, sinusitis and nervous tension. If you know your body as you should and if you are aware from day to day of your general health, there should be little reason for you not to be able to recognize and treat the cause of your headache.

While each case was individually diagnosed and treated, there was a general course of treatment used at Yungborn, to alleviate headaches. The full pack was prescribed, to be taken for á period of one hour. Cold compresses were applied during the pack. Immediately following this, the patient was bathed in luke-warm water (86 degrees). Finally, cold affusions (water jets) were directed at the head and back of the neck. In the case of the nervous headache, the affusions were also directed at the spinal column running slowly up and down the length of the patient's back. The affusions proved particularly successful. Light diets, preferably vegetarian, were also prescribed.

Zone therapy was used with amazing results in treating chronic headaches at Yungborn. I recall a woman of thirty who had suffered the pain of chronic headaches for a period of two years without relief. The woman was despondent upon entering the sanitorium and it was necessary that her condition be dealt with at once, lest she lose her sanity entirely. Benedict Lust realized this at once and acted accordingly. Demanding that the woman open her mouth., he thrust a flat metal object into her mouth and pressed upon the roof of the mouth with such strength as to almost cause the woman to cry out. Five minutes later, when the metal device (similar to an ordinary tablespoon) was removed from her mouth, the woman was unable to believe her own senses. The headache, partner to her two year misery, had entirely disappeared.

This case sighted above was not the exception but the rule as regards the alleviation of headaches. Time and again zone therapy proved the answer to this problem. The application of zone therapy in the case of headaches varied only in accordance with the area of the head affected. Where the pain was centered in the frontal area of the head, the zone pressure was applied at a corresponding point upon the roof of the mouth.

INSOMNIA

The maddening tempo of modern life, with its suicidal flight from nature, has produced a twentieth-century plague. One ailment, known only to few members of past civilizations, has become a common and constant disorder in the twentieth century. Even today, among less complex civilizations, Eskimos, Africans, Pacific Islanders, insomnia is almost unknown. But in the United States, particularly in the crowded urban areas, insomnia has reached plague proportions, with many doctors filling out those barbituate sleep-pill prescriptions as fast as their pens can write. Today drug stores have turned to the barbituates as a major source of income the way they once turned to aspirins. And the poor public consumes them as they would candy. But these "candies" carry the sting of death. National sleeping pill scandals have recently reached amazing proportions as more and more foolish souls turn to these pills for a night's sleep, never to wake again.

No pill has ever cured insomnia. No powder, capsule or tonic has ever brought permanent relief. Yes, sleep can be induced through drugs. Have you ever slept the sleep of the drugged? It *is* like having bought a small share of death. To awaken from it once is frequently a ghastly enough experience to turn you against the use of such drugs forever. The dizzy, choking numbing sensation that occurs to the awakening drugged sleeper is undoubtedly among the most horrifying of all human experiences. I cannot warn too severely against such devices.

The fact remains that only a natural existence can bring permanent relief from this modern plague. Insomnia is one of the many payments that modern man makes daily for his rejection of an existence in harmony with the laws of Nature. A return to that existence is the only completely successful means for eliminating insomnia I have ever seen practiced.

Insomnia is not a disease. It is either a reaction or accompanying symptom of disease, or it is the culmination of repeated shocks and mistreatment of the nervous system. Sleep requires relaxation. Drugs are used to induce relaxation where the nervous system will not respond to the effects of even prolonged fatigue. This unnatural means of instituting relaxation is a crutch and nothing more. Even were it not for the harmful effects of drugs, the fact of their worthlessness in producing permanent relief would be reason enough to reject their use. Only relaxation in response to fatigue can produce natural slumber.

The importance of wholesome sleep is known to all. Notice the use of the term "wholesome." There are many kinds of sleep and the value derived from them is in direct relation to the quality of the sleep, not the quantity. I have myself slept four hours of good and completely relaxing sleep and felt more refreshed upon arising than on other mornings after eight hours of restless slumber. I am certain that you have had similar experiences.

Insomnia can be divided into two categories, temporary and prolonged. Prolonged insomnia is almost: always the result of unhappiness, restlessness, a feeling of being out of step or out of place in the world. In prolonged insomnia, this restless and unhappy state can be called the disease and sleeplessness only a symptom of that condition.

The return of mind and body to a state of one-ness with the world, recognizing the pattern of the world and understanding your place within that pattern, this is the road to defeating the cause of prolonged insomnia. The chronic insomniac generally recognizes his or her restlessness through signs other than prolonged lack of sleep. But recognizing this condition will not defeat it. Knowledge itself changes nothing. Only the application of knowledge can bring change. If you are a chronic insomniac, stop saying "That's the way I am and that's all there is to it."

Temporary insomnia is a common and not dangerous condition. The causes of a night or two of restlessness are many and the degree of each cause necessary to produce a. sleepless night varies with the individual. Night noises, the screech and howl of a cat, traffic sounds, the wind, or even the dripping of a faucet may produce insomnia in some, while others are able to sleep through constant din and tumult. This is largely a matter of early conditioning. Children are natural sleepers and can condition themselves to sleep under any conditions. If as a child you learned to sleep through noisy night atmospheres, you will not be bothered by common sounds. Those who have not been so conditioned can overcome a single night of disturbing sounds through the use of ear plugs, made of a waxy substance that will not harm the ears, which can be purchased at most drug stores. Night masks, shields of black cloth, can also be purchased and will prove useful in avoiding annoying rays of light.

If your sleeplessness arises from a change in environment, a new and temporary atmosphere such as a vacation hotel, a railroad train, etc., then mechanical devices for sleep such as the mask and ear plugs are perfectly valid. But I strongly warn against the use of such devices night after night in your home. These, like the sleeping pills, become crutches without which sleep is impossible. What must be realized is that if you are unable to withstand the background noises and light of your natural sleeping environment, your home, then it is neither the noise nor the light which actually is the source of your insomnia. Rather, a condition of tension producing, an over-sensitivity to such ordinarily unnoticed things is the true cause. Again the answer to such insomnia is not sleeping devices, but what might be called a pact of friendship with the world.

Insomnia cannot be treated apart from other conditions of body and mind. Total health rules out insomnia. Therefore, strive for natural health and you will be on the road to relaxation and restful sleep. Begin now by prescribing the Fountain of Youth Cocktail for yourself daily.

Temporary insomnia, arising from momentary disturbances, is best treated in advance of bed time. When you are aware that some disturbing happening, sight or news has unnerved you, to the point where it may cost you a night's sleep, that is the time to begin combating insomnia. Once you have gone to bed, it is difficult to stop the wheels of thought from turning; they must be slowed before bed time. This is best done with a program of relaxation.

Your program of relaxation should begin at least two hours before you retire for the night. In that period of two hours, it is important to avoid over-stimulation. Exactly how you do this depends upon your individual personality. If you find reading, games such as cards, checkers or chess, or listening to good music relax you, then you will have no difficulty filling most of your two hour program for relaxation. But if you tend toward stimulating reading, or if games and music excite you even moderately, then avoid them prior to bed time. Most of all, avoid contact with work that fills your day. Don't take your business to bed with you.

Half an hour before retiring, take a final walk in the open air. This is not meant to be the kind of brisk tour that best begins your day. Walk slowly, feel the cool kiss of wind upon your cheek, do a little star counting. In other words, end your day by once more realizing your part in the great universe. Modest people seem to suffer less from sleeplessness.

When you return, prepare a warm drink for yourself. Hot milk used to be the insomniac's favorite, but this was an error in judgment. The milk did not induce sleep, the warmth did. Hot lemonade or vegetable broth will have the same effect, and may be pleasanter for many. As important as the drink is the way you drink it. Sit down in a dimly lit corner of the house and relax over your nightcap. Gradually accustom yourself to the wonderful rest that lies before you that evening. Feel yourself relaxing as you sit there. This is a moment for recalling the pleasant experiences of your life. It is a moment for warm smiles.

If you have spent your pre-bed time hours in relaxation the rest is quite simple. Just before retiring, prepare a warm stomach compress. A heating pad, with the control turned to its lowest point, will do as well. Place the pad or compress upon the center of your body, from the lower half of the chest down to the hip bones. Since it is the gentle warmth that you want here and not necessarily the healing action of water, the heating pad will do this job conveniently.

Now it is time to put your body to sleep. Starting with the toes and working your way up through the body, concentrate on each segment of your physique. Feel them deaden into total relaxation one by one, toes, heels, ankles, calves, knees and so on along the length of your frame. Do not move from one area to another until you are certain that you have felt the total relaxation of the preceding area. The first time you attempt this it may take ten or fifteen minutes. The second or third time you will find your entire body quickly falling into a state of restful repose. With this your program of relaxation is complete. Sleep is yours.

NEURITIS

This inflammation of the nerves is a common and painful condition which may affect any part of the body particularly that area which is most involved in your daily labor. Nerve cells are sensitive to a lack of Vitamin B-1 and the increase of consumption of this essential matter (provided for in the Fountain of Youth Cocktail) frequently is all the treatment needed for neuritis.

Unlike arthritis, neuritis is not caused by infection. And unlike rheumatism, neuritis does not confine itself to joint areas, its home lying anywhere throughout the body's nervous system. It is now widely realized that neuritis is frequently induced through worry, fear and despair. This is another instance of the inseparable relationship between body and mind. The treatment for neuritis may therefore begin with a better understanding of the individual and his place in Nature's pattern.

PILES (HEMORRHOIDS)

The eliminatory diet and internal cleansing was prescribed for all such conditions at Yungborn. Affusions of the rectal area for a period of fifteen minutes daily proved the most remarkable treatment of this disorder. I have known of many who have treated this condition right within their own homes with the pressure provided by the flow of water from bathtub faucets. Cold (60 degrees) high pressure affusions were directed to the rectal area during these treatments which were continued until complete alleviation of this condition was attained. The general course of treatment at Yungborn ran no more than two weeks. This is but another proof of the infallibility of Nature's care.

PROSTATE INFECTION

A painful and somewhat common condition among older men, prostate infection can generally be traced to diet deficiency and infection from waste matter retained too long within the system. "When a rational diet is observed, few cases of prostate infection will be noted. In particular, Vitamins A and C must be consumed in maximum digestible quantities. The Fountain of Youth Cocktail (on page 152) provides large amounts of both of these and, when used to fortify a rational diet, will help to overcome both such deficiencies.

The natural program for treating prostate infection, as prescribed at Yungborn, involved the non-stimulating diet, reinforced with the Fountain of Youth Cocktail and additional amounts of citrus and carrot juice. Full enemas were provided for a period of three days followed by small rectal douches daily until the condition subsided. Steam compresses (a heating pad may be used) were prescribed each evening and warm compresses during the night. Regular use of the Fountain of Youth Cocktail helped to stimulate the eliminatory system sufficiently after the first ten days and the small enemas were therefore discontinued. Air and sun bathing were considered essential in Nature's program for treatment of the prostate.

RHEUMATICS

Chronic rheumatism can be said to have caused more human misery than all the wars fought since the beginning of time. Only a person who has had his body wracked with the pain of chronic rheumatics can truly understand the truth of this statement. The dull throbbing pain that lingers day and night, intensifying during periods of cold and damp, is a mortal enemy of man and a direct product of modern man's flight from nature. Improper diet, lack of sufficient sunlight and a body that has not been hardened by Nature's agents are largely responsible for rheumatic conditions.

It is necessary to distinguish acute rheumatics or rheumatic fever from the more common ailment known as chronic rheumatism or simply, rheumatism. While rheumatic fever may cause chronic rheumatism, it is by no means the sole cause. The pain of rheumatism comes without fever and the affected joints need show no outward sign of the ailment, but are generally cold and stiff.

Rheumatism is apparently among the most deeply rooted of all human ailments. I have never seen a case of chronic rheumatism, even at Yungborn, placed on the road to recovery in less than three months. And this only with the most stringent care and self control on the part of the patient. But those months were well spent, as anyone who has been relieved of the pains of rheumatism can attest.

N. S. was a successful farmer in his mid-fifties when he came to Yungborn suffering from chronic rheumatism. The pain of his ailment had forced him to give up all but supervisory work upon his farm, and this after nearly forty years of constant and agreeable work. The discontinuance of his life's work was as much a mishap for N. S. as the pain that had caused it, for he was a man devoted to his work. Retirement at his age would not only have been wasteful and difficult for him, it would have meant an early death for a man of his vigorous and enthusiastic existence.

First step in assisting N. S. was taken at the dinner table. He was placed upon a light and completely non-stimulating diet. All spices were removed and pork was strictly forbidden. Special attention was placed upon an increased consumption of green leafy vegetables and tobacco, coffee and tea were removed from the patient's living habits.

Sun bathing, particularly the bathing of the affected areas, was prescribed. Steam baths were a daily requirement followed by a brisk wet rub of the entire body (never permitting the overheated body to become too quickly cooled). The full pack was applied whenever pain was severe and the patient was permitted to remain within the pack for two hours., Following this and a thorough drying of the body, affusions were applied. The sensitive areas of N. S.'s body could not withstand the pain of direct affusion, and therefore the jets were applied in an area immediately surrounding the center of pain.

Zone therapy was partially successful in alleviating the patient's pain and was applied quite simply. A steel comb was held by the patient in that hand corresponding to the side of his body in pain. By clenching his fist so that the teeth of the comb bit deeply into the palm of his hand and holding this position, N. S. was able to overcome his pain on repeated occasions.

Air baths and frequent wet rubs were largely responsible for hardening the patient's body to the effects of changing temperature, so often the immediate cause of rheumatic pain. But only the combination of all these was able, after three months, to bring total relief to N. S. My last view of him came several years ago as I drove away from his New Jersey farm. There, standing upon the floor of his barn, Farmer N. S. was effortlessly pitching large pitchforks full of hay high onto the second floor of the barn. I would call that complete recovery.

RHEUMATISM

This condition is frequently mistaken for arthritis, since like the latter, rheumatism settles in the joint areas of the body producing great pain and discomfort. Unlike arthritis, rheumatism is not accompanied by some body infection. Many years ago it was recognized that rheumatic conditions frequently appear for the first time during the winter or early spring. Further research indicated that during these months the consumption of citrus fruits and fresh salad vegetables was at a critical low among many people. In this way, the first knowledge of a link between rheumatism and Vitamin C deficiency was come upon.

The rational diet can prevent rheumatism. However, the correction of this condition is more involved. Once rheumatism has appeared, the Yungborn program for alleviation of this condition involves increased consumption of Vitamin C (provided in the Fountain of Youth Cocktail). Nightly warm natural baths (80 degrees) and warm compresses (heating pad) will stem the pain almost instantly. Sun bathing is particularly favorable in rheumatic conditions.

ULCERS

If you had a dollar for every person who has been "cured" two or more times of his ulcers, you would be a wealthy person — probably with ulcers. For some reason, totally unknown to me, ulcers are considered an ailment of the wealthy. (Probably by the same people who think money brings happiness). Again, if you had a dollar for all the low and moderate-income people who suffer from ulcers, you would be able to balance the national budget. Ulcers will live on any income.

Obviously those who claim to have been "cured" several times of their ulcers are really saying that the pains have been alleviated momentarily. But this is no cure. The disease cannot be cured until the cause is known and treated. Rarely is the cause of ulcers treated, but rather the effect, that hole in the stomach called an ulcer, is doused with milk, cheese, drugs, etc., and then permitted to gouge itself out and start the same painful symptoms all over again.

People who never worry do not have ulcers. People who have a knowledge of what they are doing on earth and why they must do it, also rarely suffer from ulcers. Tense,, worried, nervous and unhappy people are the prime target of stomach and duodenal ulcers.

M. K. had suffered from duodenal ulcers for eight years. He had been "cured" of them five times — before he came to Yungborn in a state of painful collapse. He left Yungborn ten days later without a trace of his ulcer. How?

M. K. was placed upon a totally non-stimulating diet consisting almost totally of fruits and vegetables and their juices. In addition to this, the patient consumed four glasses of cabbage juice each day. (Raw cabbage, sliced and reduced to juice by means of an electric liquifier.) M. K. did not respond to the use of citrus juices and these, oranges, grapefruits, lemons and limes, were removed from the diet. Aside from these, however, the patient was able to consume all fruits and vegetables in liquid form or in the steamed manner in which all vegetables should be cooked. (See Chapter 10, "Nature's Diet Charts.")

During the first five days steam (Turkish) baths were administered once a day and the full pack at night. A brisk cold water rub was prescribed each morning. At the end of the first week, the steam baths and full packs were replaced with natural (hip) baths and stomach compresses on retiring for the night. These and only these were responsible for relieving M. K. of his ulcer within ten days. However, it is to his credit that the patient has since been able to maintain superb health. Only by finally returning to a state of complete harmony with Nature, both physical and mental, was he able to overcome the root of this condition that had plagued him for eight long years. To this day, M. K. continues to drink two glasses of cabbage juice each day and he is convinced that this is largely responsible for his resistance to returning ulcers.

UNDERWEIGHT AND OVERWEIGHT

Your normal weight is dependent upon three factors: height, age and skeletal structure. Naturally the weight of the individual should alter through the several stages of life. And, quite as naturally, the amount and kind of food needed to maintain the proper weight will also vary, dependent upon the person's occupation and general activity.

To say that overweight is the result of overeating is like saying that a fire is the result of a match. Who struck the match? What caused the overeating? Overeating is not a cause but rather a result. Have you noticed how your eating habits vary when you are occupied and when you are not occupied; when you are lonely and when you are not; when you are tense and when you are relaxed? The busy, satisfied and relaxed people of the world are rarely overweight. The idle, lonely and nervous people frequently are.

When you are not occupied and feel that you should be, you eat to excuse your idleness. ("I'll do it after supper—after I have a sandwich—as soon as I'm through eating—one must eat, you know.")

When you are lonely, you eat to replace the satisfaction of

friendship. When you are nervous, you eat to forget the cause of that tension or despair. Here again is proof of the inseparability of mind and body.,

The unfortunate result of unhappiness is not only overeating, but consuming worthless., fattening foods. The act of replacing some need of mind or soul with body food is a form of blackmail. You are "buying off" the mind through ransom paid the body. Naturally this ransom must be a luxurious one. That is why the unhappy people of the world dote on chocolates, ice cream, rich cakes and the like. And here a ridiculous contradiction frequently takes place. The unhappy soul stuffs him or herself with appetite-murderers and frequently neglects the essential foods for health. Thus, contradictory as it may appear, many people are twenty and thirty pounds overweight and yet anemic, undernourished, suffering the ravages of malnutrition!

I have long realized the truth in the words "happiness is medicine." You must come to realize this too, for it is an undeniable law of Nature.

The underweight people of the world are also frequently products of a mental rather than a physical condition. You have seen the "drivers" of our world, those who throw themselves into their work without a thought to their well-being. They are frequently the victims of the "success philosophy," believing that only wealth and power bring happiness. They drive themselves and their fellow workers to the peak of production and creativity, but they usually have to be driven to the table to eat. What they eat does them little good, going through their bodies like mercury as they tear back into their dedicated labor. The man who thinks that life is all work and the one who believes it all play usually both land on the scrap heap years before their time.

I will not be foolish enough to claim that underweight and

overweight are purely the result of a mind without peace; but I will maintain that anguish, nervousness, despair and disdain for fellow humans, one or all of these, are either the cause of a major contributing factor to underweight and overweight conditions as well as to much of the physical ills of the world.

In dieting to gain or lose weight, two dangers must be avoided. The underweight person must avoid increasing his intake of calories while ignoring the basic food requirements, and the overweight must beware of haphazardly decreasing his food intake, thus depriving the body of minimal energy, bone, blood and nerve nutrients. The basic diet for all should contain some organically grown foods and a full share of all the vitamins and minerals needed to maintain a healthy body and mind. Above all, beware of the fad diets which guarantee to build you up or tear you down in twenty-four hours. These "Seven Days to Health" and "Ten Days to Beauty" programs are a fraud, at best, and a hazard to your very life, at worst.

There is no overnight diet to total health. More precisely, there *is* no diet to total health. The food you eat is but one element in the pattern of your life. The road to health does not begin with your stomach alone, or your skin or your feet or mind, but with all of these and more. The road to health is that which we pave with a life lived in complete harmony with Nature.

Chapter 10, "Nature's Diet Charts," outlines several food programs which, when added to a life in total harmony with Nature, will help to provide you with the sparkling health that should be yours. There you will find food programs designed for the underweight, overweight, as well as others. These were carefully prepared at Yungborn with the aim of providing the healthiest, tastiest and most natural food program for each person's needs. In reading through these wisely chosen diets, recall the words of Socrates, "Some men live to eat. I eat to live."

VII. YOU: YOUR OWN WORST ENEMY

IT SEEMS to be one of the commonest failings of mankind to live in direct contradiction to the simplest rules of living that will prolong life and make it a healthy one. Mainly, it is the fault of blundering ahead without thinking of the consequences. "A fool denies his errors, but a wise man learns from them." This would be a good motto for all of us. To follow it is not so difficult. We must simply stop and reexamine our way of living.

We must ask ourselves, are we our own worst enemies?

In too many cases, the answer is yes. We must be constantly watchful if we are not to lose the precious gift of health and well-being. We must judge which of our habits is injurious. At this very moment, you may be committing an error that will have an influence upon you for the rest of your life.

To know whether or not you are contributing to future sickness and stealing years from the promised span of your life, compare your way of living with these seven deadly sins of modern living.

THE SEVEN DEADLY SINS

1. Are you a tobacco addict? Do you poison your whole system — your lungs and mouth and throat, your heart and blood stream—with deadly nicotine?'

129

2. Do you drink? Whether the amount is moderate or excessive, alcohol effects your liver and kidneys and heart. Do you take, a drink as a pick-me-up without knowing that alcohol's real effect is to depress not only your brain and blood stream but every organ of your body?

3. Do you overeat? Are some of your organs being required to function at more than capacity because you will not curb your appetite? Do you deliberately put an extra strain on your muscles and bones by asking them to carry a greater weight than they were intended to bear?

4. Are you addicted to drugs of one sort or another—aspirin, alkalizers, bromides and sleeping pills? Do you reach for a 'pain killer' as soon as you feel the smallest ache or pain? If you do, you are not only poisoning your system but upsetting the balance that nature so carefully provided.

5. Do you drink coffee, tea or the cola beverages without thinking that they are crippling your nerves and undermining your health? They are drugs just as truly as aspirins or sleeping tablets even though they come in the form of a hot drink or cold, carbonated beverage.

6. Are you a faddist? Do you try all the latest pills or take unreasonable exercise or go on diets whose results are damaging to the system and may even bring death?

7. Are you a foam rubber prisoner? Are you a slave to the deep-cushioned arm chair and lazy comfort so that you cannot develop a habit of activity to produce healthful circulation of your blood stream?

If your answer to even one of these questions is yes, then you *are* your own worst enemy.

Nothing, not even nature, can replace organs or tissues which have been destroyed by poison or neglect. If you have deliberately done the things which tear down the normal functioning and balance of your system, you cannot: hope to undo the damage. By following the dictates of nature, however, you can build your body to a state of health provided that you have not gone too far along the path to destruction.

I called the seven habits sins because they work against health and life. Some of them are little more than legalized murder. Nicotine is a sure killer if enough is taken into the system. Even the daily newspapers run long articles about the dangers of sleeping tablets. People everywhere recognize that these things are dangerous. Sadly, though, the warnings go unheeded. They know but they do not act.

Horrible tales are told of some of the effects of these sins of civilization. A mystery writer kills off one of his fictional characters by injecting the nicotine obtained from three cigarettes which had been soaked in water. A set of false teeth which had been left standing in a glass of cola were turned to mush. But do people listen to them and take warning?

Scientists are constantly turning up evidence that should scare people into living a rational life. The relationship of cancer to smoking has been proven. Life insurance companies spend millions to warn Americans that overweight persons are the most likely victims of diabetes, high blood pressure, heart ailments and hardening of the arteries. The 1953 annual meeting of the American Medical Association warned that two of the worst killers, high blood pressure and coronary heart disease, were aggravated by excessive prolonged nervous tension, excessive overweight and excessive tobacco.

Blundering and short-sightedness are one thing. Sheer stupidity is another, and it can be called nothing else when people reject and ignore facts that have been established beyond any shadow of doubt. In the tobacco habit, the alcohol habit, the reach-for-a-pill-or-bromide reaction, we have the seeds of the degenerative diseases. These diseases are in no way related to bacteria or accident. Heart ailments, arthritis, diseases of the veins and circulatory system are the result of deteriorating tissues. Many people refer to them as a simple aging of the organism. All people must undergo this aging process. To all people death comes after a slow and steady loss of vitality and strength.

There is no way yet known to halt this process, but there is, equally, no reason why we should deliberately hasten it. By excesses of one kind or another, by the use of these toxic agents, we are contributing to and hastening the deterioration of our vital organs.

We know today that cancer of the mouth, lip and chest are most apt to attack people who have been excessive, or even moderate, smokers. Smoking is blamed by the scientists for many other disorders of the nose and the circulatory system. New phrases have become current in our language which attest to the spread of such ailments—smoker's throat, smoker's hack or cough.

Sometimes the connection of tobacco with disease and decay is not direct, but nevertheless it is just as deadly. Some recent investigations by Dr. W. J. McCormick of Toronto, who has done considerable research work in the field of vitamin therapy, shows the relationship between smoking and Vitamin C. He has found that the smoking of one cigarette can neutralize 25 milligrams of Vitamin C. Thus, if you have one orange for breakfast and follow it by only one cigarette, you will have lost more than half of the vitamin content. One slice of pineapple, which is also a good source of this vitamin, is almost totally nullified by the smoking of a single cigarette.

We know that Vitamin C is primarily necessary for its qualities of resisting infection. It is only a logical step to presume that a smoker, whose intake of Vitamin C is destroyed by the tobacco habit, will be more open to infection than non-smokers. This theory is upheld by a recent report from the Mayo Clinic, one of our foremost research centers. They have found that four times as many smokers contact pneumonia after an operation as non-smokers. Obviously, the ability to resist infection is much lowered if a person has not the intelligence and the mere will to survive to give up smoking.

We suggest that other experiments be made along these lines. There are some ailments which are almost certainly caused or made more severe by the tobacco habit. Emphysema is one of these. In simple words, this is merely degeneration of the lung tissue. It is a common condition as we grow older and shows itself as a shortness of breath. Through age and prolonged use, the lungs gradually lose their elasticity. It becomes more and more difficult for them to expand and contract. This happens in some degree to all people of advanced age, but for some it is a serious condition while for others it is hardly noticeable. Would it not be logical to assume that those with the severest condition are the smokers?

Recent studies have also shown that persons suffering from chronic nasal and bronchial disorders are the hardest hit by shortness of breath in their old age. This is a natural consequence of these respiratory disorders. The lungs have become abnormally distended because they have had to work beyond their normal capacity in order to overcome the defect of the other parts of the body. "When we put the known facts together, they follow a familiar pattern. `We know that smoking is the cause of many nasal and bronchial disorders and, therefore, may well be the cause of shortness of breath later in life.

Each age in history is known for its particular disease or ailment. In the middle ages, it was the plague. It was brought on by the poor diet, the long hours of overwork and poor sanitation. When we think of the seventeenth and eighteenth centuries, we associate those times with the gout. People ate little in the way of fresh fruits and vegetables. Their diet was heavy with fats. Tuberculosis was the scourge of the nineteenth century. Many factors contributed to making this the number one killer. Homes and factories were sunless and poorly ventilated. Diets were deficient in vitamins. Today the killing diseases are degenerative conditions of the heart, blood system and the brain. This breaking-down and wearing-out of the human body is, in all too many cases, brought on by the excesses and abuses of modern civilization. Tobacco, coffee, aspirin and alcohol are not merely the symptoms of our nerve-shattered age but often the direct cause of it. They destroy tissues and organs and in destroying the parts, they are destroying the whole.

These first four of the seven deadly sins are well known to all of us whether or not we are far-sighted enough to eliminate them from our lives. The three remaining, however, are not as clearly seen in their true role of killers. They are overeating, faddism a/nd the morris chair habit.

Fat contributes to every form of human decay. The number one killer of our day—arteriosclerosis (or a break down of the arteries)—is caused by fat. Fat is deposited in clumps along the inner surface of the arteries and the heart. Gradually the open channel of the arteries becomes narrowed and the blood cannot flow through them easily. This leads to scars on the heart and eventually to death.

It is estimated that the useless fat Americans are carrying around on their bodies could supply enough energy to do about one and a half billion man hours of work. Actually, this useless fat cuts down a person's ability to lead a normal, productive life. We know, for instance, that overweight people tend to be less fertile than those of normal weight. The excess weight throws out of balance all the glands of the body, including the reproductive, or sexual, glands. The hormones which the glands produce and which have much to do with our general health are produced in smaller quantities. Fat overloads the bony frame of the body and puts a strain on the joints which leads to arthritis and rheumatism. In fact, there is not one part of the body that does not suffer, directly or indirectly, from overweight.

There is only one thing to do about it. Stop overeating, We know that thousands of people go around excusing their excess weight by the flimsy excuse that their glands are out of order, that they have a sluggish thyroid. In nine cases out of ten, it is simply not true. We are overweight because we overeat. Sometimes, we overeat because we have fallen into bad habits or are thoughtless. More often, overeating is not purely physical. Just as we have seen that all diseases are conditions of both the body and the mind, so we see that often overindulgence in food is a psychological state.

We used to think that: all fat people were happy. As a matter of fact, we know now that the opposite is true. Some scientists have gone so far as to predict that they may be able to cure a good deal of mental illness when they understand more about a person's eating habits. Desire for certain foods dove-tails with a person's emotional predicament. Many people, for instance, eat more cheese and ice cream or drink more milk when they are going through a particularly bad period. Unconsciously, they are asking for security.

Everyone has noticed that some women put on a lot of extra weight after they've had a baby, sometimes right after their marriage or when they've lost a husband. It used to be argued that this was only nature, but everyone of those women was faced with a new situation in life, and the easiest way to find relief from the tensions it caused was to eat. It's a lesson most

of us learned in childhood. Hunger was probably the first unpleasant sensation we knew as babies, and we learned fast that
only food could relieve this tension. That was right and good,
but too many of us carried into our adult lives the habit of relieving tensions, any tensions, with food.

Food means comfort and security. That is the main reason
why people with emotional problems are apt to fasten so much
of their attention on food. There is the woman who is so unsure
of herself and of her husband's love, that she must have constant
proof of his devotion. What better way to get proof than to
become so fat and unattractive that only true love will accept her
ungainliness? There is the man who hates his work and
complains of headaches and backaches, of feeling too weak to
carry on. So he eats to gain strength, but the fat only makes all
his symptoms much worse, and then who can blame him when
he becomes really incapable of working?

Not all overweights go to such extremes nor are their motives
so off the track and uncontrolled. Just the tensions of frustration,
boredom, and anxiety are enough to start many people on an
eating jag, and scientists sympathize with a person who claims
he simply can't stop. Understanding what brought on the craving
for food helps some, but not much. What the person really needs
is to remove the emotional problem or, if that is impossible, to
substitute some other emotional satisfaction rather than food.

The sixth of the deadly sins is faddism. Sometimes a fad
seems to start harmlessly. The basic idea behind the 'treatment'
is a good one, but it is distorted and misused. The faddist is a
person who lives by excesses—usually he runs from fad to fad.
Perhaps one week he will lie in the sun for three or four hours.
The skin is burned painfully. Sometimes to the extent of a
second degree burn. He runs a fever, has headaches. Too fre-

quent burning of this sort is known to bring on some forms of skin cancer. What is more important, his whole system is thrown off balance. When he recovers, he swears off sunbathing and takes up yoga. He stands on his head three hours a day, fasts for weeks at a time and then wonders why his whole body is rundown and his health is. in much worse condition than before.

Actually this living by excess is a part of all the other ills of modern civilization. Certainly tobacco, in even the smallest amounts, is not good for, you, but it is the heavy smoker who suffers the most in the end. Small amounts of alcohol will cause only slight reactions in the system which it may take years to show up, but the heavy drinker will almost immediately experience the ill effects of bodily deterioration. The same is true of all the other bad habits. We are not saying that tobacco or alcohol, even in small amounts, is good. We do say, however, that excess is in the very nature of things harmful and dangerous.

Faddism has other dangers. When the faddist gets sick from exposure to the sun, people jump to the conclusion that sun bathing is dangerous and that all natural livers are crackpots. By carrying a good idea to excess, he is bringing discredit upon one of the most important factors of healthful living. To live in harmony with nature is not simply a high-sounding phrase. It means just that—harmony. There must be no excess, but a blending of all that is good. It is just as much of a mistake to eat nothing but wheat germ or drink nothing but orange juice as to dose your body with drugs and poisons. People like that are harming the progress of rational living.

The seventh deadly sin is lack of activity. How many people do you know who never stir from their chairs except to eat and sleep and work? They come home in the evening, complaining about fatigue, ready to read their papers, listen to the radio, or watch T. V. On the weekends instead of getting out in the air and sun, they lounge about the house getting more and more irritable and discontented. If this were all, it would be bad enough, but this laziness of body helps to break down the natural functioning of the system.

Exercise is necessary in order to preserve a good digestion, to make elimination natural and effective, to stir up the circulation of the blood. No system can function normally if there is a lack of appetite and, hence, of enough food of the right kinds. Constipation can bring on many other ills. We know that many cases of arthritis and rheumatism are due, in part at least, to a lack of exercise. The joints become stiff, in some forms of the disease, grow together into solid bone if they are not used constantly. Heart diseases of many kinds have their origin in the poor circulation of blood.

We must list some simple warnings.

Diet is not everything.

Water cures are not enough alone.

Air baths, if taken without equal care of diet, will not cure anything.

Too much sunlight can kill.

Massage is not a panacea.

There is only one cure-all. That is nature. All the products, agents and forces of nature, properly proportioned and regularly administered is the only way to health of both the body and the mind.

VIII.   COPPER AND ALUMINUM-
THE MENACE OF MODERNISM

W<small>HILE</small> we have reviewed some of the important ills afflicting our modern way of life, there are many other abuses. We have mentioned coffee, tea and the cola beverages, but cocoa, which is so often given children, is exactly as dangerous and harmful to the system. Patent medicines are too numerous to mention. Every year sees more and more of them thrown upon the open market where every one who has the price can buy them. It was the dangers of these medicines that, more than anything else, led to the establishment of the Pure Food and Drug Administration. Limited though its powers are, this government agency has done a good deal to protect us from some of the most harmful concoctions. Nevertheless, they are still being manufactured and their sale is enormous. The gullible public rushes to take the latest pill — that is, until a still more miraculous one *is* put on the market.

Sometimes people have to be shocked into facing facts and doing something about them. Statistics, or the art of proving the truth of a fact by citing figures, was at one time capable of stirring people to think about facts. But our modern world has become filled with statistics, with mathematical formulas for everything from atomic science to human happiness. The national budget, industrial and agricultural production figures, scientific data are presented in indigestible strings of figures, a number followed by a trial of almost endless ciphers. Our heads whirl and we cease to attach much meaning to them. Dr. Powell realized this and decided to use a more dramatic method to impress upon people the fact that disease is not merely a matter of bacteria. He publicly swallowed a vial of disease-carrying bacteria. Yet he did not become infected.

Similarly, for a world that has ignored a simple statement of facts about the danger of cooking with aluminum utensils, a farmwife provided the dramatic presentation. She filled two pots, one of aluminum and the other of porcelain, with equal "quantities of water. The water was boiled for thirty minutes and then permitted to cool. Gold fish were then placed in both pots of water. In five hours the fish in the aluminum pot were dead!

This experiment was repeated many times, but the result was always the same. Sometimes death came to the fish in the aluminum pot in five or *six* hours, sometimes in that many days. The other fish, however, lived out their normal span of time.

More formal research has been made on the effect of aluminum on the human body. Aluminum has by-products that are extremely dangerous. One of these is alum which acts as an irritant, particularly on the stomach. This in turn causes disturbances of the digestion and eliminative functions of the body. Aluminum acetate, another by-product, is a standard embalming fluid. And yet, the investigators pointed out, aluminum acetate is precisely what is manufactured when vinegar is placed in an aluminum pot. The combination of aluminum acetate and aluminum chloride, which is easily formed by adding salt to the vinegar in an aluminum utensil, is a deadly disinfectant.

When we cook in aluminum pots, a considerable amount enters directly into our blood stream and is carried to all the organs of our body. The poisonous effects pile up day after day as we eat more and more food prepared in this way. While each day's amount may be small, the total can be extremely dangerous to the health. It is believed that one of the first organs it attacks is the reproductive glands. The cells of these organs are particularly susceptible to any poisonous substance. The reproductive glands, however, are but one of a chain of glands which control most of our bodily functions. Thus, they have a chain effect on the stomach, the rate at which we convert food into energy, our nervous system, our blood stream and, eventually our heart.

Dr. Arthur Coca tells of a patient whose pulse rate jumped from 72 to 92 in a short period of time. The condition did not respond to treatment until aluminum utensils were forbidden. This experiment brought similar results in five other cases.

Cooking in pots and pans made of this material is not the only danger. It is common for a housewife to drop tarnished silverware into an aluminum pot filled with a salt solution. If any other type of pot is used, the tarnish will not be removed. If aluminum combined with salt does this, you can imagine what vegetables cooked with salt in an aluminum pot will do to your stomach.

Much research remains to be done on the effect of aluminum on food values. We know, for example, that copper destroys Vitamin C. Is the same true of aluminum? This, however, is not too important except as additional evidence. We know enough about this metal to reject its use. This will cause no hardship for there are many other materials that are perfectly safe to use. Glass, porcelain and cast iron make excellent cooking utensils, but, best of all, there are the inexpensive earthenware utensils. They were the first of all cooking utensils known to man and certainly come the closest to natural cooking.

We must not think, however, that everything that was used in the early days is automatically good for us. In this connection, there is a story which illustrates the point very well. Tom is a farmer in southern California. His grandparents traveled the dusty trail from New England to California, taking with them all the things which were in their eastern home. In his modern ranch house, there is a mingling of the new and the old. The old family coffee grinder stands close to the new porcelain electric range. Beside a row of stainless steel canisters is an antique mahogony pepper mill.

Tom is proud of those antiques, but they are not just show pieces. He actually uses them. In fact, his favorite phrase is, "If it was good enough for my father, it's good enough for me." He was twitted about this, and asked, "If candle light and an ice box was good enough for your father, why do you have fluorescent lighting and a deep freeze cabinet?"

His reply came quickly. "I never said, 'If it was *bad* enough for my father, it's bad enough for me.' "

Too many of us, having learned the value of natural living, that nature's ways are unchanging through eternity, have applied that wisdom to our lives in a totally mistaken way. The fundamental forces of life remain the same, but our environment changes. From the beginning of time, men have striven for a life of greater ease and physical benefits. This search for material welfare and more leisure in which to enjoy the fruits of our labor is a natural one so long as it does not lead us to neglect the basic need of good relationships with those around us. It need not lead us away from close contact with nature. To fight against change merely for the sake of preserving all that has gone before is as foolish as it is to fight for change merely for the sake of change.

Tom's philosophy is a good one. Retain from the past those

things which have bettered man's existence and reject those which have proven useless or even harmful. Thus, we find that some of the herbal teas which our grandparents used are still helpful today, but we know that the health charms which they wore about their necks to ward off disease were useless. We reject their errors and retain their wisdom.

Ye must learn one more thing, though, if we are to live intelligently. We must reject the errors of our own day and time. There are, each day, new forms of drugs, processed foods and health fads placed upon the market for a gullible public. People thinly they are new and untried and. rush to experiment with them. Actually, they are not new, but simply new forms of the same mistaken 'remedies'. Only the packaging and the claims are different.

What is the test? How can we decide the merits of any new idea or product? The test is simple and can be applied to all things. Does this new thing bring you closer to or farther away from natural existence?

If an electric shaver eliminates the abrasions, rashes and cuts caused by steel blades, then it is a progressive instrument. The fact that this shaver is a complex device of wheels and wires that could only have been evolved after thousands of years of human intelligence has been working toward this kind of mechanical goal does not mean that its effect is unnatural.

On the other hand, coffee is a natural product, but the effect of drinking this brew is an unnatural and poisonous one. Here a natural product causes unnatural effect. So do many other products growing freely in a natural state. Poisonous berries are found along every roadside, but we would not think of eating them simply because they were 'natural'. Intelligence and moderation are the key words.

Some people claim that the automobile is an unnatural means

of locomotion, that the idea of traveling ten or more times the average walking speed of a human being is an unnatural concept. We must learn, as always, to distinguish the bad from the good. If a man uses his car constantly for unnecessary trips, if he rides down to the corner store instead of taking a health-giving walk, then the automobile is bad. But that same car can be used to take a family out into the country, to give them the opportunity to get close to nature and all its benefits. Under those circumstances, we say that the automobile is an instrument for the good.

We must, then apply this test to all the things around us. Does it bring us closer to rational way of living or does it separate us from the good that nature supplies so abundantly? Furthermore we must learn to act as we think. To know what is right is not the same as to do what is right. If we follow the laws of nature, we are storing up health and happiness for many years to come. But we must be honest with ourselves about the effect of things about us. We must keep as our watchword the maxim, To Thine own self be true!

IX.   *YOUR FIRST ONE HUNDRED AND FORTY YEARS*

Now YOU have completed the cycle. You learned at the start that there are three keys to existence: desire, knowledge and determination. You have the desire. You were born with this and all the destructive philosophies and devices of "civilized" man could not rob you of it. The knowledge of natural existence is now yours. Though it is impossible for any one man to record all that men have experienced and learned of the art of natural healing, you have received a good introduction to so vast and vital a field of learning.

As to the determination, that is something that you alone can provide. Determination has always been born out of hope and a practical plan. Too often the hopeful are thwarted by the lack of such a plan. For that reason I have reserved the following pages as a complete and detailed plan for natural existence.

The manner in which you choose to break with your old way of life will depend upon your individual condition and the degree with which you have lived in harmony with Nature in the past. Many who have never read a book on the ways of natural existence have, never the less, lived in close contact with the laws of Nature. Others have chosen to deny even the natural truths which they have learned.

You and you alone know how well or poorly your past existence has observed Nature's plan of life. For that reason only you can decide whether to break with the old ways through a day of fasting, the eliminatory diet, the grape diet or some modification of one of these.

Let me only hold out one word of advice to you in choosing and performing this break with past excesses and errors: be wise and practical in your choice and avoid painful deprivations. Reread the sections on fasting and the eliminatory diet. Above all, do not enter into this period of self-cleansing with the notion that you are punishing yourself for past mistakes.

Once you have accomplished the process of internal cleansing to your own satisfaction you are ready to begin repairing the system. Though your body demands special care and attention distinguishing it from other systems, there are certain conditions which effect us all. For that reason I offer the following plan as a general approach to natural existence.

A Typical Day of Your New Life
Morning

Start your day with a ten minute air bath. Make certain that you provide yourself with enough mild physical activity to keep the body warm. Keep the window open but avoid chilling. A half dozen deep breaths of fresh air in front of the window will start you off with that extra bit of zip.

Finish your air bath with a brisk toweling. Now it's time for your regular morning wash-up. Don't bother putting on your shoes yet. The tile floor of your bathroom will serve to harden your feet against the aches and pains of the day. If the floor is particularly cold you needn't overdo it at first; a few minutes of barefoot walking will be quite enough to begin with.

At first approach everything with care. A break with your old life must not come as a rude shock. Try at all times to blend your past life into the new road you have taken.

Cleanse your body of the wastes that lie in the lower colon through the use of a mild enema. One cup of clear, tepid water will be sufficient to cleanse you of any normal amount of waste. Following your morning wash-up dress as lightly as the season will permit and take your sunrise walk. Use this brisk walk to prepare both body and mind for a full and satisfactory day. The fifteen or twenty minutes of your sunrise walk can be put to use in planning the events of the day while your body receives the benefit of sun and air. Breathe deeply of the morning air, for it carries Nature's own green perfume with it.

Your sunrise walk will put a keen edge on your appetite. If you have had any trouble facing the breakfast table in the past just forget it. Now your problem will be one of resisting all the demands that your eyes will make. But keep in mind that it is your stomach you are about to feed, not your eyes.

Breakfast

Your breakfast should be at least half fruit or fruit juice. It *is* a good rule to start: and complete your breakfast with fruit juice or whole fruit, at least one of which should be a citrus fruit. Here is a suitable New Life Breakfast.

> Prune Juice
> Whole grain cereal with raisins and milk
> Orange juice

Here is another:

> Prunes and raisins in natural liquor.
> One slice whole grain toast and peanut butter
> Half a grapefruit

And a third:

> Mixed tomato and carrot juice
> Half cup of yogurt and fresh fruit
> Hot lemonade.

Lunch

Begin your lunch away from the table. By that I mean prepare for your lunch with a bit of relaxation. If you work with your hands all morning, sit back and rest yourself for ten minutes before galloping into your lunch. It is just that fast paced eating habit that you want to rid yourself of.

If you work with your mind each morning then you could do with a brief walk before lunch. Just ten minutes of strolling through sunfilled streets will bring the serenity you need to truly enjoy and digest your lunch. And here are a few sample menus for your New Life Lunch.

#1

Half a grapefruit
Vegetable broth
Hard boiled egg and salad (no bread)
A medium sized apple
Tomato juice or hot lemonade

#2

Honeydew melon
Sardine and salad (no bread)
Sliced banana and raw pineapple
Grapefruit juice or hot lemonade

#3
Businessman's Special

Whole orange
Hard boiled egg, whole tomato and radishes
Tomato juice, mixed nuts and raisins

You are used to the practice of washing your hands before

each meal. Now I ask you to practice washing your mouth after each meal. It is not necessary that a toothbrush be used, though this is the most effective method. Just a few mouthfuls of water rinsed in the mouth to loosen any bits of food that may continue to cling after your meal will help protect your teeth against decay. It's a simple habit and one you can easily adopt.

Afternoon Tone-Up

Before rushing back to work you'll do well to clear your head with an afternoon tone-up. This doesn't require a gymnasium and ten thousand dollars worth of equipment. Just two minutes of your time will do the trick. Start by pulling your shoulders back and taking a half dozen deep breaths of air near an open window. Now relax your shoulders. Now pull them back again. Repeat that a dozen times. Now tilt your head back and close your eyes. Place the palms of your hands gently over the eyes and rest for half a minute. That's all. Simple? Of course. Worthwhile? Try it and see for yourself.

Dinner

On your first day you must attempt to avoid large amounts of protein and starch. In advancing from a fast or eliminatory diet into a first day of natural diet you must not tax your system. This warning is particularly well taken in the matter of your evening meal.

For most of us the evening is the least physically active part of the day. Why then is the evening meal so often the biggest, starchiest, most dedicated to energy foods? This seems to be another of those up-side-down habits that we have gone along with for years without questioning. Here are some suggestions for *rational* evening meals at the beginning of your natural life.

#1

Vegetable broth
Cottage cheese salad
Sliced bananas and pineapple
Orange juice or hot lemonade

#2

Tomato and celery juice
Tuna fish salad
Mixed fruits*
Coconut milk or hot lemonade

*Dried apricots, prunes, figs and raisins which have been soaked overnight in water with a small amount of raw sugar added to taste. Make enough of this delicious fruit mix to last a week. Be sure all dried fruits are unsulphured.

#3

Spinach and carrot juice
Cheddar cheese, chopped eggplant and salad
Sliced apple, orange and pineapple
Grape juice or hot lemonade

Natural Bath

Evening time presents the best opportunity for your natural bath. Taken before retiring, there is less opportunity for your body to become chilled following the bath. In addition, the luke warm bath water will create the kind of mood that best supports a good night's sleep.

Immediately after your natural bath is a fine time for your regular body inspection. This does not have to be a daily event. However, frequent and regular body inspection is the best kind of preventive medicine. It is these regular check-ups that will help you to discover minor and major abnormalities in their first stages. Be on the lookout for any unusual skin discoloration, lumps, bruises or wounds. Report to your physician any of these which persist for a week or more.

Odds and Ends

Weighing yourself should be included in your regular evening check-ups. Any abnormal loss or gain of weight should also be reported. You should weigh yourself at least once a week.

Many persons find this time of the day best suited for their daily bowel movement. Of course, the important thing is not the time of day you choose, so long as you set aside a particular hour and make this a regular part of your schedule. Simply by providing a particular time for this vital function and maintaining that schedule, you will soon create a condition of regularity.

Changing your bowel habits is not a difficult matter and the benefits derived from it are well worth the effort. Many people who suffer from constipation do so simply because they can not comfortably use the strange toilet facilities of their place of work, and they have not bothered to train themselves to evacuate only during an hour when they are in their own homes.

Twilight Time

This is the moment when your night's sleep will be decided. Once you have climbed into bed and begin to wrestle with your pillow it is too late to prepare for sleep. The time to relax body and mind is before you have entered your bed. A warm glass of milk, fruit juice or lemonade is a good beginning for a fine night's rest.

Now, glass in hand, sit down in a comfortable chair and relax. Turn some of the lights out and sit in the semi-darkness with a few idle thoughts and kind memories of the day. Some deep breathing is all the exercise you'll need. Fifteen minutes of relaxation is a good road to slumber land. Now open the windows wide, check to make sure that you have enough bedcovers and climb into bed.

The opening days of your new schedule should follow approximately the above outline. Each succeeding day will permit you a fuller menu but you will never again return to that poor mixture of starches and sweets that you once called "food".

By the fourth day you are ready to consume greater amounts of nutrition. Time then to begin drinking your Fountain of Youth Cocktail. You may like to start and finish your day with the cocktail. Certainly the most convenient and suitable times of the day for it are mid-morning and mid-afternoon.

Fountain of Youth Cocktail

This should be made in a liquifier, not in a juicer. Cut up and put in the following ingredients: 4 oz. pineapple juice

3 large celery stalks
2 carrots
4 tablespoons of dry skimmed milk
6 almonds
2 tablespoons of wheat germ
6 apricots (pitted, dried, unsulphured if fresh are unavailable)
6 prunes (pitted, dried, unsulphured if fresh are unavailable)
2 medium sized oranges (peeled)

Add enough water to make liquid the proper consistency to drink. Where the system will not easily accept citrus fruit, as in the case of ulcer sufferers, substitute 1 fresh red pepper or 2 green peppers for oranges.

About ten thirty in the morning and three o'clock in the afternoon, when the business of the day has begun to sap some of your energy, take a ten minute break. Have a glass of the Fountain of Youth Cocktail and a little munch to go with it. Here are a few suggestions.

Snack # 1

Mixed nuts and raisins

Snack #2

Sunflower seeds and two prunes

Snack # 3

A tablespoon of peanut butter and teaspoon of wheatgerm

Snack # 4

A tablespoon of yogurt with some fresh fruit

Snack # 5

One carrot and tablespoon of cottage cheese

Snack # 6

A whole tomato and teaspoon of wheatgerm

Fruit juices need not be chilled to be enjoyed. If you prefer them cold, however, and cannot obtain them where you work, buy a thermos bottle and take them to work with you.

Though each succeeding day will permit you to extend your diet until you have reached a well balanced food schedule, there are certain rules which should prevail from the start.

Always undercook your vegetables to gain all their values.

Include some organic food in your daily diet. (Sunflower seeds, squash seeds, sesame seeds, etc.)

Eat a diet; as close to the natural condition of the foods as possible. This means fresh foods uncontaminated with poisonous sprays and preservatives and prepared with a limited amount of seasoning.

Use imagination in preparing your meals. Good meals need not be dull and unappetizing. On the contrary, unappetizing meals can't be good for you no matter what the table of food values may say. Try a new food each week. To get the most out of eating enjoy what you eat.

Sun, Earth and Water

Employ your natural surroundings to the advantage of your health and welfare. Provide for sunbathing and barefoot walks whenever possible. Seriously consider building yourself a sun-hut someplace nearby that you can get to at least on weekends if not daily. Or find a nearby solarium, swimming pool or open air gymnasium.

If you own your own home put some chairs outside in a slightly shaded area and do as much working and playing out there as you can. Take your shoes off on weekends as often as possible.

Remember the word of warning about sunlight. Too much sun is as bad as arsenic and twice as painful. Take your sunlight through the trees or cover yourself with moistened leaves. Don't bathe immediately before sunning yourself or you'll lose some of the vitamin D.

Try sleeping out on warm evenings. At the very least, spend part of your weekend lying on the ground. Let your body once more feel that happy surge that comes with earth contact.

Water cleans internally as well as externally. Don't reserve the internal wash for periods of illness. A weekly enema will keep the lower colon free of waste and serve to tone up your entire system. Let the enema do for your internal body what the natural bath does for your external body.

Housecleaning

Here's your housecleaning list. See to it that none of these darken your closets again. Keep these slow-poisons as far from you as possible: refined sugar, bleached flour, processed cheese, cocoa, coffee, tea, alcohol, tobacco, colas and other carbonated drinks, aluminum utensils, aspirin and other drugs, deodorants.

X.   NATURE'S FOOD CHARTS

ARE YOU attempting to get life from dead foods? In recent years more people have come to realize the importance of selecting the foods that will most benefit their health. This interest in the life-giving values of food is good and marks here a great advance in human welfare.

EAT ALL FOODS AS CLOSE TO THEIR NATURAL STATE AS POSSIBLE

Most food is overcooked. What is more, many people have the habit of peeling vegetables, potatoes in particular. They should never be peeled for the most valuable elements lie directly under or in the skin.

PASTEURIZATION

Pasteurization is the process of boiling milk at some 145 degrees Fahrenheit for the purpose of destroying disease bacteria. The process was named for Louis Pasteur who discovered that boiling wine at a certain point in its aging process would destroy the bacteria which might; otherwise turn it into vinegar. Since that time pasteurization has been credited with protecting the entire human race against destruction. This is unadulterated nonsense.

It is possible for a sick cow to transmit certain diseases to humans. We must guard against this by only using milk obtained from healthy cows. The government has employed many examiners for many years now to examine all cows whose milk is to be sold and certify that the animals are not infected, particularly to insure that they are not tubercular. This wise policy now assures us of disease-free milk. Then why pasteurization? If the milk we drink is already proven safe for human consumption, why is it necessary to boil it before it may be sold?

Pasteurization not only kills disease germs, but it also destroys the bacteria which sour milk, just as Pasteur originally destroyed the microbes which turned wine to vinegar. Thus, by boiling milk for a specified time, it is possible for the large milk companies to guarantee that the milk may be stored for several days without spoilage. The little farmer and the small local dealer were never concerned with this problem, since they sold their milk but a few hours after it left the cow. This is the reason that the large milk companies pasteurize and it is the reason why they have fought for the laws demanding pasteurization.

Pasteurization would not confuse most people as to its value if it had a more obvious name—if, for instance, it were simply called "boiling." Most people know what boiling does to food values. Vitamins are devitalized or totally destroyed by boiling. In particular, vitamin C is sensitive to heat and much of this anti-scurvy vitamin is lost through pasteurization. This is of extreme importance to parents who are attempting to protect or rid their children of scurvy and its ravages upon teeth, bone and blood.

In addition to its lower vitamin content, cooked milk is far less easy to digest than raw milk. For this reason many doctors prescribe raw milk for sensitive young stomachs; more would do so if it were possible for raw milk to be obtained everywhere. The milk trusts have done such an excellent job of driving raw milk off the market that it is totally impossible to buy truly fresh milk in many areas. If you live near a farm there is no problem. It simply means that you must buy your milk from the farmer before he delivers it into the hands of the pasteurizers. If you don't live within reasonable distance of a direct raw milk source, it would be worth your while to search for a store or market which carries it. In California, the most health-conscious state in the nation, it is quite easy to obtain raw milk; and I am told that in many areas, particularly new communities with young families, raw milk actually outsells the pasteurized product. Each day more people have come to realize that pasteurized milk is a fraud, created to foist old and devitalized milk upon the nation.

DON'T USE SODA TO ADD "GREEN" TO VEGETABLES

There are two dangers here. Soda destroys the vitamin content of food, and it reacts on aluminum to produce poisonous substances which enter your blood stream.

GET YOUR VITAMINS AND MINERALS NATURALLY. DON'T RELY ON "ENRICHED" AND "VITAMINIZED" PRODUCTS.

Nature has provided an abundant supply of vitamins and minerals in foods in their raw state. If you have not destroyed them by peeling or overcooking, you will receive an adequate supply so long as you eat a rational diet. The so-called enriched foods have already been devitalized. The mere addition of a chemical equivalent of the necessary vitamins and minerals does not compensate for the loss of natural food elements.

USE SALADS IMMEDIATELY AFTER CUTTING OR SHREDDING THE VEGETABLES

The Vitamin C content of vegetables is lost at an extremely fast rate once the vegetables fibres have been cut or bruised.

DON'T THROW AWAY THE WATER USED TO COOK VEGETABLES

Drink it, or save it for tomorrow's soup. Such water is rich in the vitamins extracted from the vegetables during the cooking process.

DON'T SKIP MEALS TO REDUCE

Your body requires regular and frequent supplies of energy. In reducing your weight, it is not how much or how often you eat that counts, but *what foods you choose* and how well you chew them.

EAT A GOOD BREAKFAST

Coming as it does at the start of a new day and after fourteen or more hours without nutrition, breakfast is a means of replenishing your energy and strength. It will help carry you through some of the busiest and most demanding hours of your day. If you want to reduce, choose a salad instead of a heavy meal at lunch time, but only after eating a nourishing, balanced breakfast.

HAVE AN AFTERNOON PICK-ME-UP

A glass of Fountain of Youth cocktail at three or four o'clock will serve as that extra boost to help you get through the remainder of the day.

EAT SOME ORGANIC FOOD EACH DAY

Include at least one food that is organically grown in your daily diet. It would be ideal if all the fruits and vegetables we consumed were organically grown, but there are not enough organic farmers to supply us with all our needs. The next best thing *is* to include at least one food that has been organically grown. Those most easily obtained are pumpkin, squash and sunflower seeds. They will provide the final link with natural nutrition which each of us must maintain.

COOK VEGETABLES QUICKLY AND IN VERY LITTLE WATER

The value of food which is created in the growing process is easily destroyed in the process of cooking. All foods should be cooked far less than is the habit in most homes today. Very often the water in which they are cooked is more valuable to your health than the vegetables themselves. You should eat your food in the state closest to its natural condition.

It is necessary to know three things about the cooking of each vegetable. How long should it be cooked? How much water should be used? Should the pot be closed or open during the steaming? For this reason, I have prepared the following table to guide you in building a diet that will remain rich in vitamins and minerals.

VEGETABLE COOKING CHART

VEGETABLE	AMOUNT OF WATER	POT	COOKING TIME
Asparagus	2 inches	closed	10-18 minutes
Beans, lima	2 inches	closed	16-28 minutes
Beans, snap	2 inches	closed	10-20 minutes
Beets	1 inch	closed	16-20 minutes
Beet greens	1 inch	closed	6 minutes
Broccoli	1 inch	closed	12-20 minutes
Brussel sprouts	1 inch	closed	6-8 minutes
Cabbage	1 inch	closed	6-11 minutes
Carrots	1 inch	closed	12-20 minutes
Cauliflower	1 inch	closed	12-16 minutes
Chard (leaves)	1 inch	closed	6 minutes
Chard (stalks)	1 inch	closed	12 minutes

Corn (on cob)	1 inch	closed	4-8 minutes
Dandelion greens	cover veg.	closed	6 minutes
Kale	cover veg.	closed	12-16 minutes
Parsnips	cover veg.	closed	13-25 minutes
Peas	cover veg.	closed	8-13 minutes
Potatoes, white (medium)	cover veg.	closed	20-25 minutes
Potatoes, sweet (medium)	cover veg.	open	25-30 minutes
Spinach	cover veg.	open	5 minutes
Squash	cover veg.	open	6-8 minutes
Tomatoes (quarter)	cover veg.	open	8 minutes
Turnips	3 inches	open	16-25 minutes
Turnip greens	dry	open	13-16 minutes

Now for the most important task of all, learning the nutritional value of most of the commoner foods. If you understand the contribution each food can make to your well-being, you are equipped to devise a sensibly balanced diet for yourself and your family. All the foods referred to are fresh — not canned, frozen or preserved.

APPLES: This fruit is particularly rich in minerals, especially if eaten raw with the skin left on. They are also excellent in eliminating constipation for they contain a good deal of water and cellulose.

APRICOTS: This fruit ranks immediately behind liver as a source of iron. They should be a regular item on your shopping list because they can do much to build and replenish your blood supply.

ASPARAGUS: Particularly useful in increasing and controlling body elimination. Recommended for reducers, asparagus contains the vitamins and minerals most useful in fighting off infections.

AVOCADO: This is one of the most complete foods in vegetable form. They contain a rich supply of protein, but they are also the fattiest of all vegetables and so should be avoided by those wishing to reduce. They are a fair source for infection fighting, eye-nose-and-throat aid and clear skin vitamins.

BANANAS: This fruit has been somewhat maligned by those who warn against it; as being highly fattening. Bananas are a medium calorie food and have even been recommended, coupled with milk, as a reducing diet. This combination, eaten without supplementary greens, however, is a very unbalanced diet for they lack many food essentials. They are very helpful in the treatment of kidney and stomach ailments and have been used with remarkable success in the treatment of sprue and "celiac stomach" (intestinal indigestion), disorders quite common to children.

.But it is important to· remember that bananas are not beneficial if unripened and may be a cause of indigestion. Look for the brown specks that indicate ripeness when purchasing bananas. If your stomach is sensitive to foods with concentrated amounts of roughage, prepare them with a liquifier. Many wonderful desserts can be made by blending bananas with other fruits and with cream cheese. A blend of pineapple and banana is particularly delectable and nutritious.

BEANS: All the beans, with the exception of green (snap) and yellow (wax) beans, are closely related nutritionally. Kidney, soy, lima and navy beans are all good sources of protein. Baked in tasty casseroles, they can be substituted for meat or fish. All, again with the exception of snap and wax beans, are high calorie foods and should be avoided by those who are overweight.

Kidney beans are a good source of Vitamin B-1 (energy) and have relatively good amounts of riboflavin that is an aid to clear skin. Sensitive digestive systems may require that kidney beans be put through the liquifier. Soy beans are good energy and clear-skin food. Soy bean sprouts are high in infection-fighting value and may be used as a vegetable or as a tasty salad ingredient. Lima beans, both green and dried, are an excellent food. Dried limas are fine sources of energy and elements for clear skin. In a casserole and accompanied by a salad and a raw fruit dessert, dried limas make a good and inexpensive meal. Sensitive digestions may not accept dried limas easily. Preparation in the liquifier will help in digesting them. Green limas, though not as good a source of B-1 and riboflavin as the dried bean, contain a higher degree of value for the eye-nose-throat and are high in mineral content. They make an excellent substitute for potatoes. Navy beans are a wonderful energy food and a fair source of clear-skin aid. Like green limas, navy beans have a good share of minerals. Baked with molasses, tomato sauce, etc., navy beans are a tasty treat. Snap beans and wax beans, unlike those listed above, are low in protein and an excellent choice for reducers. They are valuable in promoting the health of the eye-nose-throat and are a fair source of infection-fighting.

BEETS:

High in natural sugar, they provide a good source of body fuel. Not a particularly valuable food, their appetizing tang makes them a good addition to any balanced meal. I heartily recommend beet soup (borsht) topped with a tablespoon of sour cream or yogurt as a genuine taste thrill. Served cold, it is a summer-time delight.

BEET GREENS: A very valuable food! Beet greens are an extraordinary source of eye-nose-throat aid and clear skin value. It is also of great value in enriching your blood with iron and manganese. Recommended for reducers.

BLACKBERRIES: Successfully used in treating dysentery. Should be prepared in blender if digestion is a problem. Good reducing food.

BREAD: Whole grain breads are an excellent source of minerals and the B Vitamins. White bread and all that made of processed flour are nearly valueless arid serve to add calories without other services to the body. Various forms of preservative and bleach used in these breads are harmful to your body and mind. Where sensitivity to foods high in roughage causes you to avoid whole grain breads, cooked cereals may be more easily digested. It is possible to receive the minerals and B Vitamins required through nut butters and wheat germ preparations that can be made with the aid of a blender. Wheat germ and nuts can also be blended with fruit juices which may assist your digestion of these valuable foods. Bread is high in caloric content and should be eaten sparingly by reducers.

BROCCOLI: A valuable vegetable rich in value for the eye-nose-throat and clear skins and for fighting infection. A good bone builder, it contains large amounts of potassium which is necessary for proper growth and the health of heart and nerves. Overcooking makes broccoli less digestible.

BRUSSEL SPROUTS: Contains fair amounts of elements necessary for the eye-nose-throat, clear skin and fighting infections. Good reducer's choice. As in broccoli, avoid overcooking to aid digestion.

BUTTER: Its food value varies with the season and the quality of the butter. A good source of vitamins for the eye-nose-throat and for bones. It also provides you with essential acids. Evidence indicates that butter should be avoided by those sensitive to skin disturbances (fats are believed to be a contributing factor in acne and other skin disorders) and in cases of gall bladder infections. Overheating butter (frying) destroys much of its food value

CABBAGE: Good infection fighter. Green (Chinese) cabbage is good source of eye-nose-throat aid. The vitamin content is best preserved when it is served raw. Sliced raw cabbage should be eaten fresh and not made in large quantities for storage since exposure tends to dissipate Vitamin C.

CARROTS: Excellent. eye-nose-throat aid. Make carrot juice a part of your diet each day. High on list for reducers and older persons.

CAULIFLOWER: It is an aid to clear skin and infection fighting. The green leaves are especially helpful in fighting infection and make a tasty salad addition. Steam cauliflower for a short period of time to preserve the vitamins.

CELERY: Use green, not white, celery. It contains moderate amounts of elements for the eye-nose-throat. Celery consome (steam chopped celery for three to four minutes) is an excellent aid to digestion. Celery leaves are particularly valuable and should be used in salads, sandwiches, soups, coleslaw, etc.

CEREALS: Whole grain cereals are recommended to increase Vitamin B intake. Whole bran is injurious to the digestive and eliminatory systems. Fair protein source but not recommended for overweights.

CHARD: This too-little used vegetable is an excellent source of eye-nose-throat aid and rich in iron. Wonderful food for reducers.

CHEESE: A good meat substitute and an excellent source of calcium and phosphorous. Cottage cheese, because of its low caloric content, is particularly recommended to reducers. Cream cheese, on the other hand, is good for those wishing to gain weight. Processed cheeses, with their dangerous preservatives and high water content, are strongly warned against.

CHERRIES: Rich in copper and manganese, they are recommended for blood building. Fair source of infection fighting and eye-nose-throat aid. Acceptable for reducers when eaten in small quantities.

CHOCOLATE: Contains theobromine, closely related to the deadly caffeine. Useless for any purpose other than adding weight. May also cause skin eruptions, particularly among the young. All cocoa products contain theobromine and should be avoided.

COFFEE: Valueless and destructive. Avoid coffee completely. Substitute milk, cereal coffees or, if necessary, caffeineless coffee.

COLLARDS: Fine value for energy, eye-nose-throat aid and fighting infections. High calcium (bone building) content with good share of potassium, iron and phosphorous. This is a *must* for every diet.

CORN: Rich in iron and copper, it is a good eye-nose-throat aid and infection fighter. "White corn has little value for the eye-nose-throat. It should not be eaten by those with sensitive digestive tracts. Always eat it in combination with a green vegetable or salad which will balance its vitamin deficiency.

CREAM: Contains a good share of necessary fatty acids. Good eye-nose-throat aid. Should be avoided by reducers because of its fat content.

CUCUMBERS: Not vitamin-rich, but it contains erepsin which is of great value in aiding digestion. Eat with the skin if this can be easily digested. Include cucumber in two meals each day if you are bothered by poor digestion.

DATES: High mineral content, particularly iron, potassium and magnesium. Should be avoided by overweights and employed by underweights.

EGGPLANT: Fair amounts of infection-fighter and B Vitamins. Excellent food for reducers. High amount of roughage.

EGGS: Protein content equal to that of organ meats. Rich in all minerals and B vitamins. Highly recommended for blood poverty. Good breakfast food, containing stable amounts of energy. Eaten raw, blended with milk or fruit juices, eggs will supply you with necessary iron. Hard boiled eggs are easily digested. One egg a day is a minimal amount of this precious food.

FIGS: Good laxative quality, rich in iron and B Vitamins. Fine substitute for unnatural sweets. Not recommended for reducers.

GARLIC: Increases the appetite when served in salads at beginning of meal. Strong reason exists to consider garlic of antiseptic and anti-bacterial value. Little food value.

GELATIN: High protein value when consumed in strong solution (one tablespoon of powdered gelatin to one-half glass of water). May be found useful in treatment of stomach ulcers. No vitamin value.

GRAPEFRUIT: Fine source for energy and fighting infections. Low caloric content. Excellent for reducers. Grapefruit juice may be digested by those who cannot easily assimilate orange juice. Useful in treatment of colds and influenza.

GRAPES: Excellent kidney stimulus. Believed to be useful in treatment of various allergies. Low in vitamin value and may be difficult to digest.

KALE: Tops in eye-nose-throat aid. Good clear skin aid and infection fighter. High amounts of iron, calcium and potassium. One of the best of all foods for reducers. Eat kale twice a week at the very least.

LEMON: Good in treatment of colds, influenza and fevers and excellent for fighting infections. Good for reducers, but they should not be eaten raw from the skin as this is believed to have a destructive effect upon the teeth.

LENTILS: Rich in minerals and protein. Good energy aid. Should not be eaten by reducers.

LETTUCE: Green leafed lettuce better than white. Romaine and chicory are excellent sources of clear-skin, eye-nose-throat aid and for fighting infections. Useful in balancing system against allergies. Highly recommended for reducers.

LIMES: Good as infection fighter but not as good as oranges or lemons. This low calorie fruit may be more easily digested than other citrus fruits. Make certain that your diet includes one citrus fruit each day to protect your body against infection, mouth diseases, fatigue, scurvy and joint pains.

MARGARINE: Does not contain animal acids found in butter but even those margarines fortified with Vitamin A have not been completely proven the equal of butter. Not recommended for children.

MELONS: Cantaloupe contains good amounts of elements to fight infections and aid the health of the eye-nose-throat. Also some B Vitamins. Casaba and honeydew are not as vitamin rich. Watermelon good for fighting infection but not much eye-nose-throat protection. May produce gaseous-ness in those with such a tendency. Recommended for reducers.

MOLASSES: Excellent source of iron and therefore a must in the diet of all anemics or potential anemics. (Here the term anemia is used to refer to iron deficiency.) Should be substituted for sugar and candy. Contains B Vitamins. Combined with whole grain and flour, molasses will produce tasty and healthful baked goods.

MUSHROOMS: Rich in B Vitamins. Fine vegetable for reducers.

NUTS: Good protein value. Good source of B vitamins. Difficult to digest. Not recommended for reducers and forbidden to gall bladder patients.

OKRA: Successfully used in treatment of stomach ulcers, particularly when juice or broth is made with liquifier. Fair amounts of eye-nose-throat aid and clear-skin value.

OLIVES: Little food value, but tasty addition to your menu. Not recommended for reducers.

ONIONS: Like garlic, onions are believed to have an antiseptic or antibacterial quality. Young onions are more healthful than the large, white kind. They are an excellent source of eye-nose-throat aid and good for fighting infections. Onion sandwiches have been reported as successful treatment for insomnia. Onion broth (quickly steamed) is a delicious dish and has been used for many years as a treatment for head colds.

ORANGES: Excellent for fighting infections. Large quantities of orange juice should be consumed during fever, rheumatism and gum disorders. Can be drunk by reducers without too much fear, but raw fruit is better than juice for reducing purposes. Oranges are the most valuable of all citrus fruits and should be a part of your every-day diet.

PARSLEY: Excellent vegetable, containing high amounts of Vitamin A and C and several minerals. Use liberally in salads, soups, etc.

PARSNIPS: Fair source for energy and fighting infections. Good choice for reducers. Rather high in roughage.

PEACHES: Yellow peaches (fruit coloring) a fine source of eye-nose-throat aid. Highly recommended for increasing hemoglobin count in the blood. Dried peaches are also valuable.

PEANUT BUTTER: Excellent source of B Vitamins, making this a fine energy food. Should be shunned by reducers. A mixture of wheat germ and peanut butter makes an excellent spread and offers even greater energy value.

PEARS: Good bowel stimulant. Vitamin and mineral content not extremely high, but a good food for reducers.

PEAS: Dried peas offer a rich supply of minerals and protein. Should be used sparingly and those who tend toward gaseousness. Fresh peas offer an even richer source of energy and a fair amount of eye-nose-throat aid. Rich in sodium and potassium.

PEPPERS: Fine source of eye-nose-throat aid and good for fighting infection. Use in salads, sandwiches, coleslaw, etc. Find as many uses as possible for fresh peppers as they are a valuable addition to your diet.

PICKLES: Useless. Pickles are forbidden for acid conditions.

PINEAPPLE: Delicious fruit. Fair source of infection fighter and energy. Fresh pineapple is suitable for reducers but canned pineapple is heavily sugared and nutritionally less valuable after canning.

PLUMS: Good aid to digestion. Recommended for reducers.

POTATOES: White potatoes are a fair source of energy and for fighting infection if their vitamins and minerals have not been peeled and cooked out of them. Never peel potatoes. Scrub and cook in their jackets. Sweet potatoes are an excellent source of eye-nose-throat aid, but they contain a substantial number of calories which makes them forbidden fruit for reducers. White potatoes are not so fattening. Reducers may eat one medium-sized potato each day without fear. But not butter, margarine or gravy!

PRUNES: Rich in many minerals. Excellent food for blood building. Fine for maintaining bowel regularity. Do not stew prunes, apricots and raisins if you wish to retain vitamins.

PUMPKIN: Good source of eye-nose-throat protection. Recommended for reducers if eaten without sugar.

RADISHES: Good vegetable for reducers. Fair for fighting infections. Radish tops (about one inch of greens) should be used in salads, soups, etc., as they are even more valuable than the radish itself.

RAISINS: High iron content makes the raisin an excellent food for anemics. Also highly alkaline, helpful in overcoming acid conditions. A splendid blood building salad consists of raisins, prunes, avocadoes and carrots. This is not recommended for reducers, however.

RASPBERRIES: Good food for reducers with fair infection fighting value.

RHUBARB: Most valuable as an aid to digestion, but does not contain high vitamin value.

RICE: White, polished rice is practically useless and only serves to add calories. Brown rice is a good source of energy and an aid to clear skin. Rich in calories.

SOUPS: Soups made of vegetables that have not been overcooked contain most of the rich vitamin values of those vegetables. Soups are a good meal starter since the warm liquid tends to ease the tensions of the day and place the eater in a relaxed frame of mind.

SPINACH: Excellent source of eye-nose-throat aid. A fine food for reducers. Spinach should be a regular part of your diet and may be served lightly steamed as a vegetable, raw in salads or mixed with other cooked vegetables or eggs.

STRAWBERRIES: Fine source for fighting infection. Good for reducers. May be more easily accepted by the system if steamed for sixty seconds.

SUGAR: White sugar is useless and endangers human health, causing tooth decay, stomach fermentation, excess fat, etc. Brown sugar is little more useful. Raw sugar has mineral values not contained in the refined products and is recommended for all purposes.

TANGERINES: Good source of energy, nose-eye-throat aid and for fighting infection. May be found more digestible than oranges.

TEA: Useless and as destructive as coffee.

TOMATOES: Fine eye-nose-throat values and fair quantities of elements for energy and fighting infections. Excellent food for reducers.

TURNIPS: Turnip greens are far more valuable than turnips alone. These greens are among the richest in eye-nose-throat protection as well as a good source of clear-skin aid. Turnip greens have a very individual flavor that may not be immediately acceptable to some. If these greens are sliced and blended with other vegetables before being quickly steamed, they may be found more acceptable. It is important that you find the most enjoyable means of preparing turnip greens since they can be of such great benefit to your health. Turnips, though less valuable than their greens, are recommended as an anti-allergy food.

WATERCRESS: Good source of eye-nose-throat aid and fair amount of clear-skin protection. High amount of roughage. Excellent food for reducers. Serve watercress often with salads.

WHEAT GERM: Excellent source of B Vitamins which will help protect you against cataracts, dim vision, skin eruptions, heart and nervous disorders. Good source of phosphorous.

YEAST: Among the finest of all sources for the B Vitamins. Where diet restricts your intake of bread, wheat germ and other cereal products, a daily quota of yeast should be added to your diet to fulfill your requirements for energy, clear-skin aid and to fight pellegra.

I hope that this table will serve to clarify some of the questions about nutrition that have long puzzled you. Maintaining a balanced diet is not a difficult task once you understand the value of each food and your own individual requirements.

Sometimes you have asked how your daily diet should be changed to overcome certain specific ailments. I am listing below some of the more common ailments and the dietary treatment best suited for each.

DISEASE	DIET
Anemia	Up to a week on all-fruit diet followed by two to three weeks fruit and milk diet. (Start with two pints of milk daily and gradually increase

Anti-Fatigue and Blood Building

to four or more pints.) The follow Nature's basic diet recommended later in this Chapter.

Where fatigue arises from dietary deficiencies, place special emphasis upon the following foods: nuts, cheese, butter, and beans. Four glasses of Fountain of Youth Cocktail each day will add most of that extra spark you require. As already mentioned, a salad of raisins, prunes, avocadoes, and carrots proved effective in combating fatigue

Asthma

produced by anemia. Short fast regime followed by ten to fourteen days on a restricted diet, then Nature's basic diet, (Short fast and restricted diet should be repeated at intervals of two months, as necessary,

Arterio-Sclerosis

for the time being.) Seven to ten days on all fruit diet, then Nature's basic diet. Two or three days on ail fruit diet four weeks from time normal diet

Bladder Disorders, Prostrate Enlargement, etc.

is begun. Same treatment as Colitis.

Blood Pressure (High)
Bright's Disease (Kidneys)

Same treatment as Arterio-Sclerosis Short fast regime. Then fruit and milk diet for two to four weeks. (Further fasts and periods on fruits and milk if necessary.) Then Nature's basic diet.

Bronchitis (Acute) symptoms	Complete fast until acute have disappeared. Then all fruit diet.
Bronchitis (Chronic)	Short fast regime followed by ten to fourteen days on a restricted diet. Then Nature's basic diet. (Further periods on short fast and restricted diet at intervals if necessary.)
Catarrh (Chronic)	Five to seven, ten, or fourteen days on all fruit diet. Then Nature's basic diet. Occasional shorter periods on all fruit diet from time to time.
Clear Skin	Fortify Nature's basic diet with extra amounts of peanut butter, beans and dried peas, wheat germ, bananas and eggs.
Colitis	Short fast regime followed by ten to fourteen days on a restricted diet. Then Nature's basic diet. Further periods of short fast and restricted diet if necessary.
Constipation (Chronic)	Seven to fourteen days on all fruit diet, then Nature's basic diet. Occasional shorter periods on all fruit diet if necessary
Colds (Acute)	Twenty-four to thirty-six hours fast on orange juice. Then two or three days' all fruit diet
Colds (Habitual)	Same treatment as Catarrh
Diabetes	In early stages, short fast regime followed by fruit and fruit and milk diet very beneficial, if no insulin

	taken. Individual physician's advice essential *in all cases,* however.
Diarrhoea	Twenty-four to thirty-six hours' fast on orange juice. Then milk diet for as long as necessary. Five to seven or
Dyspepsia (Nervous)	ten days on all fruit diet, followed by fruit and milk for a further week or two, taking up to four pints of milk daily. Then Nature's basic diet. Occasional further periods on fruit and milk, if necessary. Short fast, ten
Ear Troubles (Catarrhal Deafness, etc.)	to fourteen days on restricted diet, then Nature's basic diet. Further periods on short fast and restricted diet will be necessary at intervals.
Eczema (Also Psoriasis and Dermatitis)	Short fast regime. Ten to fourteen days on restricted diet. Then Nature's basic diet. Short fast and restricted diet to be repeated at intervals as needed.
Epilepsy	Short fast. Restricted for fourteen days. Then Nature's basic diet. Repeat short fast and restricted diet at intervals.
Fevers (Scarlet Fever, Smallpox, Typhoid, Diphtheria, Pneumonia, Measles, etc.)	Fevers of all kinds should be fasted completely until abated. Then gradually go through all fruit and fruit and milk diet to Nature's basic diet. Same treatment as Indigestion.
Flatulence (Also Heartburn)	
Gastritis (Acute)	Complete fast for two or three days. Then all fruit diet until well again.

Gastritis (Chronic)	Same treatment as Chronic Indigestion.
Goitre (Also Graves* Disease)	Short fast. Restricted diet for seven to fourteen days. Then Nature's basic diet. Further periods on short fast and restricted diet if necessary later. Short
Gout	fast regime followed by restricted diet for ten to fourteen days. Repeat short fast and restricted diet at intervals of two months, if necessary.
	One to ten days on all fruit diet each
Heart Disease	month. Follow by further few days on fruit and milk diet. Then Nature's basic diet.
	Twenty-four hour's fast. Then all fruit
Indigestion (Acute)	diet for two or three days. Five to seven days on all fruit diet, followed
Indigestion (Chronic)	by a week or longer on fruit and milk; or short fast regime and ten to fourteen days on restricted diet. Then Nature's basic diet. Further periods on fruit and milk, or further fasts and periods on restricted diet at intervals, as necessary. Seven to ten days on all fruit diet, then Natures'
Liver Disorders (Biliousness, Jaundice, etc.)	basic diet. Two or three days on all fruit diet every fortnight if necessary.
	Same treatment as Rheumatism. Five
Lumbago Neurasthenia	to seven days on all fruit diet.

	Ten to fourteen days on fruit and milk diet, starting with two pints daily and increasing to four or more. Then Nature's basic diet. Further periods on fruit and fruit and milk at intervals, if necessary. Same
Neuritis	treatment as Rheumatism. Nature's
Overweight	basic diet with these exceptions: Remove two slices of bread, all starchy vegetables (except for one baked potato every other day) and sweet fruit juices. Substitute whole citrus fruits for citrus juices. Use skimmed milk and non-fat beverages. No nuts or nut butters. Eat a piece of fresh fruit or one glass of Fountain of Youth Cocktail mid-morning and mid-afternoon to appease hunger.
Piles	(See Chapter IX.)
Pyorrhea	Short fast. Restricted diet for ten to fourteen days. Then Nature's basic diet. Further periods on short fast and restricted diet at intervals.
Quinsy or Tonsillitis	Fast until acute symptoms have disappeared. Orange or pineapple juice may be taken every two hours. Then all fruit diet followed by fruit and milk.
Rheumatism and Arthritis	Seven to ten or fourteen days on all fruit diet. Then Nature's basic diet. Two or three days on all fruit diet

Sciatica

Skin Diseases
  (Impetigo, Urticaria,
  Acne, Eruptions of all
  Kinds, etc.)

Tumors

Ulcers (Gastric or
  Duodenal)

Underweight

every month from then on. If severe, short fast, fourteen days on restricted diet to begin with instead of all fruit diet, with further fasts and periods on restricted diet thereafter, at intervals, if necessary. Same treatment as Rheumatism. Seven to ten or fourteen days on all fruit diet, followed by period on fruit and milk if necessary, then Nature's basic diet. Occasional further short periods on all fruit diet followed by fruit and milk from time to time if necessary.

Short fast. Restricted diet for fourteen days. Then Nature's basic diet. Fast and restricted diet to be repeated at intervals if necessary. Short fast. Fruit and milk diet for two, three or more weeks. Then Nature's basic diet. Short fasts and periods on the fruit and milk diet may be necessary in certain cases. Nature's basic diet with special emphasis on cereals and whole grain bread, nuts and nut butters, dried dates and figs particularly when served in cream cheese or salad dressing, and daily serving of avocado. Drink four glasses of Fountain of Youth Cocktail each day with crisp soy crackers or roasted nuts. Milk,

	cream and dairy products should be liberally eaten,,
Varicose Veins	Seven to ten days on all fruit diet. Then Nature's basic diet. Further short periods on all fruit diet from time to time.
Worms	Seven to ten or fourteen days on all fruit diet followed by fruit and milk diet for a period. Then Nature's basic diet. Further periods on all fruit and milk diet later if necessary.

Unlike the diet charts of the faddists, Natural diets are all constructed around a basic food program to which additions are made in accordance with the aim of the individual. This basic diet must supply all the natural food requirements. The theory that overweight people can live off the energy which they have stored in their fatty tissue is both false and dangerous. Few vitamins can be stored within the body. They must be obtained each day from the food we eat. This requires a central balanced food program for all.

Again, unlike the faddist, the natural diet should not be a written and memorized procedure. I have outlined the values contained in most of the common foods so that you will be able to judge their worth for your personal diet. Once you have understood these values it will never be necessary for you to follow a written schedule. You will now be able to choose your foods individually and intelligently with a view to sound health and fitness.

RETURN-TO-NATURE DIET

Before establishing the basic natural diet which will afford you a lifetime of healthful nutrition, you must first cleanse your system of years of waste. The thousands of meals of processed foods, of fatty meats and of overcooked, valueless vegetables have all taken a toll upon your body. Before anything else, the body must be cleared of the sludge that has been left behind by these dead foods.

A cleansing period of two weeks was found to be the time required by the average patient at the sanitoria. A low calorie and milk protein diet was devised to wash the system and return it to the natural state from which point health and happiness could be reconstructed. When combined with a daily small enema and herbal laxative pills, the cleansing process is complete.

This Return-to-Nature diet was provided not only for those who showed serious disrepair, but for all who came for treatment, no matter how mild the apparent illness. All too often sickness exists for years without giving an outward sign that we can detect and then suddenly erupts from within you. It *is* for this reason that some ten years ago I made it a rule to place my · self upon the Return-to-Nature diet for a period of two weeks, four times a year, regardless of my outer signs of health, I have never regretted this decision.

Breakfast: Citrus juice, a dish of dates, figs and prunes and a glass of skimmed milk. (The dried fruits should be steeped in water overnight, not cooked.)

Lunch: Salad, consisting of carrots, raw cabbage, raisins and a choice of one of the following: tomatoes, onions, celery, chives, dill, watercress, peas, string beans or asparagus. The last three vegetables may be steamed for several minutes to aid digestion. A vegetable oil and lemon dressing may be used to add zest to this bowl of health. Two small portions of steamed vegetables complete this meal. A glass of fruit or vegetable juice will finish off the luncheon but should not be drunk during the meal. Any excessive amount of liquid during a meal serves to dilute the gastric juices within the digestive system and increased difficulty in digestion may result.

Dinner: A salad of fruit and cottage cheese, half and half, using any or all of the following: apricots, prunes, raisins, apples or peaches which have been soaked overnight. Make sure you drink the fruit water, too, or use it as a dressing for the salad. If you tire of the cottage cheese, eat the fruit salad and follow it with a cup of pea soup (no meat stock) or add a serving of ripe bananas to the salad.

It was the rule at Yungborn to permit the patient himself to decide at what point he wished to add to this Return-to-Nature diet. Generally, at the end of a week, improvement was noticeable and the patient felt eager to increase his life-giving diet. At that point, a steamed or baked vegetable was added to the evening meal and, if the improvement was marked, one or two slices of whole grain bread were added to the daily diet, a slice at breakfast and one at lunch, none at the evening meal.

I would regard it as a foolish gesture to attempt to rebuild natural health without first discarding the poisons and waste matter of unnatural existence. For that reason I consider the Return--to-Nature diet to be step one in your new life. Once having cleansed your system, step two, Nature's Basic Diet, lies ahead of you, with its promise of good eating and good living.

NATURE'S BASIC DIET

Three servings of high protein food each day. You may select from the following: eggs, wheat germ, yeast, nuts and nut butters, dairy products (particularly non-processed cheeses such as Roquefort, cream cheese and natural cheddar), cereals and certain vegetable casseroles (lima beans, kidney beans, lentils and dry split peas).

One serving of citrus fruit each day.

One fresh salad and two servings of steamed vegetables or vegetable juice each day, the total of which will include at least one of each of the following groups:

Group A: Potatoes (white), brussel sprouts, chives, collards, dandelion greens, kale, mushrooms, parsley, spinach. Group B: Mustard greens, turnip greens, watercress, beet greens, chard (leaves and stalk), collards, dandelion greens, endive, escarole, kale.

Group C: Carrots, turnip greens, spinach, collards, dandelion greens, beet greens, mustard greens, sweet potatoes squash and kale. Group D: Cabbage cauliflower, tomatoes, peas, spinach.

Four slices of whole grain bread each day.

Fresh or dried fruits daily, particularly apricots, peaches, cantaloupes, dates and figs.

A daily serving of dairy products.

A daily serving of vegetable oil (salad dressing or bread spread), particularly olive oil, soybean oil or peanut oil.

This is Nature's basic diet. This combination of citrus fruit, vegetables, whole grain bread or cereal, fruit, dairy products and vegetable oil is the basis of a sound diet. Enriched with at least one organically grown food and two glasses of Fountain of Youth Cocktail, this schedule forms a perfect diet for all human beings.

The work now being done on dietary therapy each day uncovers new and amazing knowledge of the healing powers which Nature has deposited in the fruits of the soil. But you do riot need the most recent laboratory information to know how and what to eat. Avoid all processed and devitalized foods and make fruits, vegetables and nuts a major part of your regular diet. Eat at Nature's table and live the full promise of life.

INDEX

INDEX